Mommy, I'm Hungry!

Also by Jeanne Warren Lindsay
(Partial listing)

Your Baby's First Year
El primer año de tu bebé
The Challenge of Toddlers
Teen Dads: Rights, Responsibilities and Joys
Teenage Couples — Expectations and Reality
Teenage Couples — Caring, Commitment and Change
Teenage Couples — Coping with Reality
Pregnant? Adoption Is an Option
Do I Have a Daddy? A Story for a Single-Parent Child

Also by Jeanne Lindsay and Jean Brunelli
Your Pregnancy and Newborn Journey
Tu embarazo y el nacimiento de tu bebé
*Nurturing Your Newborn: Young Parents' Guide
to Baby's First Month*
Crianza del recién nacido

By Jeanne Lindsay and Sally McCullough
Discipline from Birth to Three

By Jeanne Lindsay and Sharon Enright
*Books, Babies and School-Age Parents:
How to Teach Pregnant and Parenting Teens to Succeed*

Mommy, I'm Hungry!

Good Eating for Little Ones

Jeanne Warren Lindsay, MA
Jean Brunelli, PHN
Sally McCullough

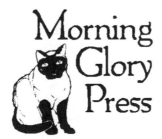

Morning Glory Press

Buena Park, California

Mommy, I'm Hungry!
is part of a seven-book series. Other titles are:
Your Pregnancy and Newborn Journey
Spanish - *Tu embarazo y el nacimiento de tu bebé*
Nurturing Your Newborn
Spanish - *Crianza del recién nacido*
Your Baby's First Year
Spanish - *El primer año de tu bebé*
The Challenge of Toddlers
Spanish - *El reto de los párvulos* (2007)
Discipline from Birth to Three
Spanish - *La disciplina hasta los tres años* (2007)
Teen Dads: Rights, Responsibilities and Joys

Note: The "regular" editions of the above titles are written
at sixth grade reading level.
Your Pregnancy and Newborn Journey, Nurturing Your Newborn,
and *Your Baby's First Year*
are also available in easier reading editions
which test GL 2 using the Flesch Grade Level Formula.

**Library of Congress Cataloging-in-Publication data
available upon request.**

ISBN 978-1-932538-54-0, cloth; 978-1-932538-51-9, paper

MORNING GLORY PRESS, INC.
6595 San Haroldo Way   Buena Park, CA 90620-3748
714/828-1998   1/888-612-8254
email info@morningglorypress.com
www.morningglorypress.com
Printed and bound in the United States of America

Contents

Preface

We (Jeanne, Sally and Jean) have worked with teen parents for a total of 72 years. We have had many many wonderful students who parented their children beautifully.

However, we were concerned when we saw infants and toddlers being given foods that wouldn't help them develop as well as they could. Sometimes a mom would give her infant solid food before his digestive system was mature enough to handle it. Before he was a year old, a child might be fed French fries and other fast foods. Toddlers were sometimes labeled picky eaters, and some apparently would eat little more than cookies and fruit drinks or soda.

These mothers, you understand, were doing what they thought was best for their children. Perhaps they weren't especially interested in nutrition. Or perhaps they weren't very knowledgeable about the importance of giving their child healthy foods.

Of course it's not only very young parents who fall into this pattern of providing poor food choices for their children. Older parents often are in the same situation.

This is why we decided to write this book. We aren't suggesting that you and your children should never eat fast foods. We aren't saying you should spend hours in the kitchen following elaborate recipes for every meal. We are saying that if you choose foods from the various basic groups — fruits and vegetables, dairy products, whole grains, and protein foods — and add only a small amount of junk or fast foods occasionally, your child will be healthier now, and will be less likely to fight the battle of obesity when s/he's a teenager.

Note: While the title is *Mommy, I'm Hungry!* this does *not* mean it's written only for moms. Dads can and often do play an important role in guiding their children toward the healthy foods they need.

We hope you, both moms and dads, find this book interesting and useful.

Good eating to you and your family!

Jeanne Warren Lindsay
Jean Brunelli, PHN
Sally McCullough

Foreword

I am excited to see ***Mommy, I'm Hungry!*** — a new book on nutrition for young parents and their children. Nutrition education is essential for quality prenatal care and feeding of young children. However, guidance is frequently limited or inadequately addresses the special needs of very young mothers and fathers.

Information in this book is also useful for the extended family as they support the young parents in selecting healthy foods for themselves and the baby.

One of the most impressive aspects of this book is that food and nutrition needs, a subject in which many young people are not interested, is discussed in practical, easy-to-understand terms. The young mothers' individual stories speak directly to other teens to reinforce positive eating practices for both pregnant mothers and their young children.

Nutrition guidelines are presented chronologically from pregnancy to preschool years of the child with added chapters on food shopping and easy-to-make food recipes for young children. However, a frustrated mom with a toddler that is a picky eater could go directly to that chapter for help without having to read the beginning chapters.

The book's down-to-earth approach includes several topics generally not found in a book on nutrition. These topics include an explanation of differences between serving and portion sizes, discussion of vegetarian diets for pregnancy and children from infancy to preschool, and tips on shopping for healthy food within one's budget.

Good food choices during pregnancy provide the building blocks for the fetus to grow and develop into a healthy baby. This book is a valuable learning tool as it includes discussion on teen challenges such as eating fast-food and avoiding obesity.

The USDA's MyPyramid is the food guide followed throughout the book. Using MyPyramid, rather than food fads, to plan meals will ensure that foods are providing necessary nutrients.

Mealtime for infants and all children is very important. It not only provides nutritious food for good health but is a time for infants to bond with mom and/or dad and the child-care provider. It is an opportunity to develop family rituals such as everyone eating as a family at the table rather than in front of the television.

One of the best gifts for a new baby is for mom to breastfeed as long as possible, preferably for a year, according to the American Academy of Pediatrics (AAP). Breast milk has the right amount of nutrients needed for the baby's growth and development, is easier than formula for newborns to digest, and has antibodies to help infants fight infections and diseases.

Breastfeeding is also good for mom. It not only saves time and money but it will help in losing pounds gained from pregnancy!

The authors consider the problems facing a young woman who must return to school or work, yet knows her baby needs to be breastfed. If she attends a school with childcare on campus, this should be no big problem.

If baby cannot come to school or work with mom, the authors point out that moms can pump their breasts two to three times daily and immediately store the expressed milk in the refrigerator. The expressed milk can then be taken to the childcare provider for the baby's feedings the following day.

They also note that expressed breast milk gives Dad or grandparents a chance to feed the baby occasionally.

Good resources for assistance with breast-feeding problems include La Leche League and the Special Supplemental Nutrition Program for Women, Infants, and Children (WIC).

Because of individual circumstances, some mothers choose to bottle-feed their baby. Formula that is iron-fortified is sufficient for the first six months. By this age, the baby needs additional nutrition and is ready to learn about solid foods.

The family's attitudes, likes/dislikes of food, and cultural/ethnic food practices will influence the baby's eating habits. In *Mommy, I'm Hungry!* the authors describe techniques for introducing new foods, observing cues for hunger and fullness, preparing home-made baby foods, and identifying foods that are choking hazards for babies and toddlers.

As the baby moves into the toddler stage, she will be ready to drink from a cup, eat finger foods such as teething biscuits (*not* French fries!), and small amounts of table food that have been chopped, mashed, or pureed.

Encouraging a taste for vegetables and coping with a

"picky" eater are discussed. It's important to remember that a toddler's portion is much smaller than that of an adult.

If Mom and Dad regularly eat fast food, sugary cereals, and sodas, the child will demand the same foods. This is likely to lead to a preschooler who is overweight, needs dental care, and has developed poor eating habits which could negatively impact his body for some time.

Being overweight is a concern at any age. It is particularly bad for a child as he may be teased, have physical or emotional problems, and be at high risk of becoming an overweight adult.

A study released in September, 2006, by the Institute of Medicine indicates that one-third of the children and youth in the United States are obese or at risk of becoming obese. Over the past 30 years the obesity rate for children aged 2-5 years has tripled to 14 percent, making childhood obesity a growing public health concern in this country.

The first battleground in the war on obesity begins at home. Habits that will reward children with good health include eating breakfast, consuming nutritious foods, getting appropriate exercise, avoiding excessive time in front of the television or playing video games, and limiting empty calorie foods.

Following the Food Pyramid for Kids guidelines found in *Mommy, I'm Hungry!* will help parents plan and serve nutrient-rich meals to young children. By participating in physical activity such as chase and dance, family members and the children, even very young ones, will get large muscle exercise and burn calories.

Every day millions of people opt for a quick, cheap meal at a fast-food restaurant. We are surrounded by fast-food messages both at home on television and in the community where restaurants are on many street corners. The lure of inexpensive food, not having to cook, and perhaps that free toy for the kids is hard to resist.

Few people stop to consider the nutritional value of the food for themselves and their children.

The authors don't insist that all fast food is bad. Instead, they offer examples of fast food menus that provide no more than a fourth of the individual's daily calorie, carbohydrate, fat, and salt needs. They write, "We aren't telling you all fast food is bad. We are suggesting you make good choices when you do eat fast foods."

Young mothers attending school or going to work are faced with childcare issues. Maybe grandmother is available or perhaps childcare is provided as part of the school program. Whatever the choice, the young parent needs to consider the options in terms of what is best for the child.

I was privileged to work with pregnant and parenting teens in a school program for eleven years and at the California State Department of Education for fourteen years. Many pregnant students in my school-based program entered with poor and irregular eating habits that were insufficient not only for their own nutritional needs but compromised the health of their unborn child.

The young moms often were surprised to learn that many foods they planned to let their children "taste" such as French fries are inappropriate and/or dangerous.

This experience was invaluable when I had the opportunity to develop public policy at the state level for a comprehensive program for these young people. The outcome was the California School Age Families Education (Cal-SAFE) Program, a state-funded school-based program designed to increase availability of support services for expectant/ parenting students and provide child care/development services for their children.

One of the required support services is the provision of nutritional supplements to the pregnant moms.

To use the subsidized child care service, the parents
must participate in parenting education. Here they learn
about nutrition and healthy eating practices for their
children and themselves.

Additional information on Cal-SAFE is available on the
Web, **<http://www.cde.ca.gov/ls/cg/pp/>**

The authors of this book, Jeanne Warren Lindsay, Jean
Brunelli, and Sally McCullough, together have over 60
years of working closely with pregnant and parenting teens.
From this extensive experience, ***Mommy, I'm Hungry!***
reflects their knowledge, sensitivity, and insight into these
young people and the challenges they encounter.

Mommy, I'm Hungry! is a significant tool for learning about nutrition and good health during pregnancy
and about appropriate diets for children from infancy to
preschool. Of course the book can be used by itself or in
conjunction with other instructional strategies.

In addition to the young mothers themselves, ***Mommy,
I'm Hungry!*** is a tremendous resource for educators,
health care practitioners, social workers, childcare provid-
ers, and grandparents for supporting pregnant and parenting teens in implementing quality dietary practices. The
community of professionals working with these youths will
appreciate this excellent addition to Morning Glory Press'
large body of resources written especially for this
population.

Ronda Simpson-Brown, Lead Program Consultant (retired)
Cal-SAFE Program, California Department of Education

Acknowledgments

First of all, we want to thank the young parents whose comments add so much to this book. Talking with each one and hearing them express their love and concern for their children was a joy. These young people include Alejandra Castillo, Amanda Lachica, Amber Flick, Angenique Graves, Anjelica Marchese, Autumn Hannold, Axciriz Palma, Breanna Wallace, Brenda Ortega, Crystal Melendez, Donna Cruz, Gladys Medina, Heidi Chavez Vazquez, Jerica Pacheco, Jessica Boutelle, Jessica Hayes, Jessica Pyper, Julianna Kostar, Kayla Kaiser, Kayla Lane, Latisha Sherman, Marcia Mann, Maria Flores, Maria Negrete, Mayra Calderon, Mayra Durazo, Myina Rodriguez, Nicole Arnold, Nicole Caston, Patricia Cruz, Robin Lewis, Samantha Gibson, Shardá Harris, Siera Huff, Tuesday Boyd, Valeria Maldonado, Whitney Burkett, and Yesenia Herrera.

These delightful young parents were referred to us by teachers and others from around the United States. We deeply appreciate their help. They include Judy Gustafson, Darlene E. Yoquelet, Helen Richards, Betty Ann Morton, Bob Gross, Peggy McNabb, Laura Barhydt, Laura Severson de la Torre, Shirley

Swartwood, Deberra Grazier, Julie Tolman, Pat Bohannon, Pepi
Baker, Josephine Cravalho, Theresa Arnold, Renee Radicella,
and Heidi Sauvey. If we've left anyone out, please forgive us.

We especially want to thank the generous people who advised
us and/or critiqued our manuscript. Juanita Weber, director of the
California School Age Families Education (CalSAFE) program,
provided wonderful support. Ronda Simpson-Brown, formerly
lead program consultant of CalSAFE, wrote the Foreword. We
appreciate her. We thank Becky Escoto for her comments con-
cerning group childcare. We thank Mary Shimer, R.D., for help
in locating information about vegetarian diets.

Others who read the manuscript and offered suggestions
include Vicki Lansky, Diane Smallwood, Martha Roper, Glen
Jacobson, Pati Lindsay, Dee Jacobson, Marilyn Simpson, Betty
Overley, Julie Tolman, and Lola Jane Collinge.

Angela Allen-Hess and Shirleen Larson organized the photo-
taking for photographer Colleen Magera. Sam Westcott and Erin
Lindsay provided two of the photos. Jami Moffett is responsible
for the lovely drawings.

Tim Rinker designed the cover, and Steve Lindsay critiqued
the layout of the book.

Eve Wright did lots of proofreading and generally kept Morning Glory Press alive and well during this time. Thank you, Eve!

Mike Brunelli and Stuart McCullough provided plenty of love
and support during our book writing. Daughters Sue Brunelli
Leas and Evelyn McCullough Reitz supplied some of the recipes
and tips in the last chapter. And last, I, Jeanne, want to thank Bob
in memory for his support of past books. He would have liked
this one, had he lived.

Jeanne Warren Lindsay
Jean Brunelli
Sally McCullough

*To the teen parents
we have known and loved,
who give so much that their children
may have satisfying, healthy lives.*

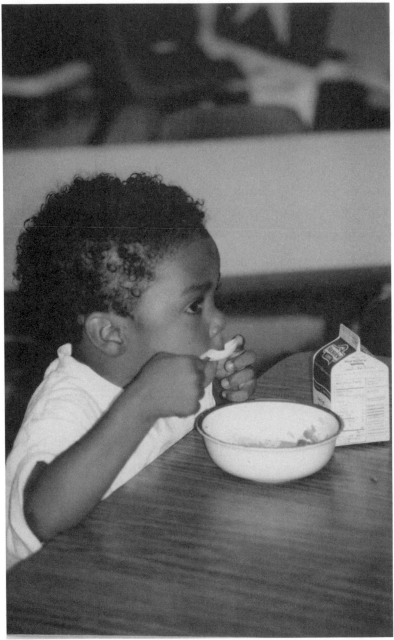

What he eats now has a big influence on his health through the years.

Introduction

Moms and dads should be role models for their babies. If the baby sees you eating fast food, junk food, he'll get that habit. When you want him to eat good food, he's not going to want to – he'll copy you.
Dolores, 18 – Enriko, 21/2

We don't have soda in our house, never. We don't buy it, and we rarely drink it.

There was a time when I did, and it's amazing how much weight you lose when you quit drinking soda. It's kind of weird if that's all you do to lose weight.
Hannah, 23 – Mackenzie, 41/2

What You Hear

You've probably grown up with television ads bombarding you constantly. "Eat this and you'll be gorgeous." "Choose this fast food and you'll find love." "Smart people drink this brand."

Now your child is seeing the same constant, attention-getting advertising of fat-laden fast foods, sugar-filled soda, and cereals that contain little more nutrients than candy. You take her to the store with you and she demands this cereal and that drink because TV said she should get it.

Not only must you cope with heavy advertising on most children's TV shows, but you may also find a fast food restaurant on nearly every corner in your community. And who wants to cook when you can buy French fries, double bacon burgers, and soda that easily?

So what's a parent to do?

You want your child to be healthy. You don't want him to be overweight now or when he's a teenager, or ever, for that matter.

You don't want him to run the risk of the illnesses that can result from poor nutrition, such as diabetes and asthma. But in our culture, it's a real challenge to meet those goals for your child.

Hopefully, this book will help you help your child learn to eat the foods that will give her a chance at a satisfying life as the healthy person you want her to be.

We talk a lot about nutrients. A nutrient is a "nutritious substance" according to the dictionary. Regularly consuming foods high in the key nutrients is an extremely important part of keeping our bodies healthy.

The six key nutrients are vitamins, minerals, protein, carbohydrates, fat, and water. We need generous amounts of most of these nutrients. However we should limit the fats and sugars in our diet and in our children's diets.

Making Good Choices

Of course we have chapters suggesting good food choices for the various stages between conception and age five. We consider separately the needs of pregnancy and the breastfeeding mother (because that's how a child is best fed between conception and six months), the baby aged 6-12 months, the toddler, and the preschooler.

We aren't simply discussing the foods you and your child need at various stages. We also have a chapter focusing on fast foods. (Yes, you *can* make healthy choices at most of the fast food restaurants, but it takes good planning and determination on your part.)

Another important chapter shares various tips to help you help your child avoid obesity. You may find these two chapters especially interesting.

We also discuss planning a healthy vegetarian diet, and

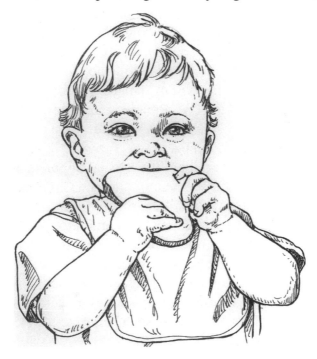

on food needs in childcare centers.

Do you live with your parents or your partner's parents? If you aren't responsible for the food that's served in your home, it may be a little more difficult to make the changes you might like to make in your child's eating habits. Communication with your extended family may be the key. Perhaps you will share some of these suggestions on teaching babies, toddlers, and preschoolers to enjoy a wide variety of healthy foods. If you decide you and your child need to cut back on the fast foods you eat, you may want to ask your family for support in doing so.

Resources for More Information

Research on nutrition is constantly updated. You will probably find articles in your newspaper telling you about new discoveries, how this specific food or that one will do wonderful things for your health. These articles are not always good resources for deciding what to eat. And television ads for food certainly are not!

Throughout the book we have followed guidelines for good nutrition from the USDA (United States Department of Agriculture) and their MyPyramid model for daily food choices. MyPyramid for Kids is reproduced on pp. 99-100, and for adults, pp. 49-50.

Have you signed up for WIC (Special Supplemental Nutrition Program for Women, Infants and Children)? If not, call your Public Health Department for information. You may be able to get coupons for certain foods you need for yourself and your child. If you're a teenage mother, this may qualify you for help from WIC.

A pilot study was recently done by WIC that allowed coupons for buying fruits and vegetables. Federal regulations may be changed to allow such purchases. Check with your WIC office.

Note to Newcomers to the United States

Many families who are new to the United States may find it challenging to continue the well-balanced diet they followed in their native country. In urban areas there may be many specialty markets for groups of people looking for their customary diet. In other parts of the country, especially in smaller communities, this may not be true.

Children in newly arrived families, just like most children, are influenced by American television and advertising, which creates a second challenge. We hope this book can help these families continue their tradition of good nutrition for themselves and their children.

We focus more on traditional American foods here, knowing we can't possibly do justice to the food preferences of everyone. The basic message — we all need foods from each of the basic food groups — applies to all of us. However, the specific foods preferred from one family to another will vary.

Shopping, Cooking with Your Child

Good, healthy food can be expensive. One chapter offers tips to help you plan your food shopping to include the foods you and your child need, while keeping within your budget.

The last chapter is a mini-recipe section. If your child helps you cook, he's likely to want to eat the food you two prepare. You'll find some recipes for simple, good-tasting, and healthy snacks, quick lunches, and main dishes, plus a couple of desserts.

As you read, you may relate to some of the young parents who are quoted, as they share their challenges and successes with promoting healthy eating for their children.

Good reading and healthy eating!

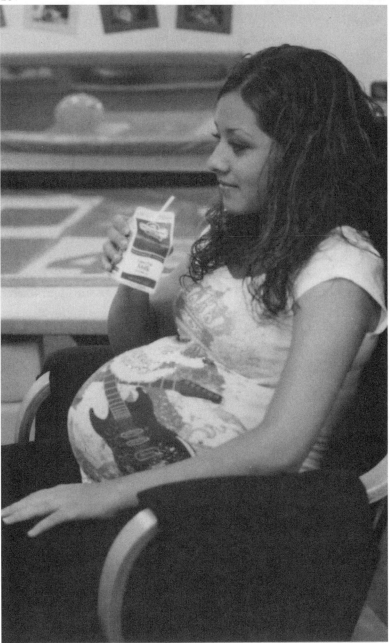

She's providing the good food her unborn baby needs.

1

Feeding Your Unborn Child

- **Eating Right During Pregnancy**

- **Follow This Guide**

- **First, Milk or Other Calcium-Rich Foods**

- **More Protein During Pregnancy**

- **Fruits and Veggies, Whole Grains**

- **So What's a Serving?**

- **Read the Labels!**

- **Making Good Choices**

I tried to eat really healthy while I was pregnant. I knew what I ate during pregnancy would affect my baby.

While you're pregnant, stay away from the sweets. Make sure you eat your vegetables, like the ones that are real colorful. They have more good stuff in them.

Drink enough milk because that affects your bones.

Don't overeat! Just because you're pregnant doesn't mean you have a license to eat everything you want.

Monique, 18 – Ashley, 5 months

I had to see a nutritionist because I had an eat-ing disorder before I got pregnant. I was bulimic and anorexic. She gave me a big list, things I could and couldn't eat. I changed how I ate a lot. I always took my vitamins.

I'd make myself an egg in the morning and a piece of toast. I'd try to eat salads for lunch, and drink those shake things that give you more nutrition. Then I'd eat whatever my grandma cooked at night.

I've always had a problem eating meat, but I'd force myself to eat it because I wasn't doing it for myself. I was doing it for my baby.

Cynthia, 17 – Julian, 11 months

Like all parents, you probably have dreams about your baby even before s/he's born. How will your baby look, feel and act? Happiness, healthiness and fitting into the world are all values you want for your upcoming family.

You have the power to affect those things before your child is born. One of the most important ways you can do that is by eating well. You want to provide good nutrition for both yourself and the child within you.

The information and suggestions included here can help you make choices that will result in the happy, healthy, thriving child of your dreams. No matter how far along you are in your pregnancy, you can make changes today that will benefit both you and your baby.

Eating Right During Pregnancy

I changed what I ate when I was pregnant — a lot more salad, oatmeal, lots of bean and alfalfa sprouts. I craved good food.

I didn't even want anything sweeter than fruit. No chocolate cake!

Lauren, 20 - Makayla, 15 months

Why does nutrition matter? What difference does it make whether or not you eat the foods you and your baby need? Here are some excellent reasons:

- **Helps you gain the right amount of weight for you and your healthy baby.**

    I was way overweight before, and I gained 40 pounds. Baby was only 3 pounds, 13 ounces. She was born six weeks early because I had pre-eclampsia.

                                                                    Monique

For most women, 24-26 pounds is recommended. However, if you're a pregnant teen, and you're still developing, you may need to gain more, perhaps as much as 35 pounds.

If you were overweight or underweight before you became pregnant, that can also affect how much you should gain. Ask your healthcare provider for specific help. You want to know what's best for you and your baby.

- **Prevents high blood pressure and toxemia (eclampsia)**

    I got toxemia, so Pancho was delivered at 35 weeks by C-section. When I was pregnant, I drank a lot of soda, one or two cans a day — 1 1/2 liters a day.

    Sometimes I crave sweets, but I don't eat a ton of chocolate. By six or seven months I wanted to eat all the time. I fixed smoothies. I'd get the smoothie mix and add whatever fruits I wanted, generally bananas and strawberries, plus mango and papaya. I ate about every two hours. I gained 35 pounds.

                                                Querida, 18 – Pancho, 10 months

One of the most serious complications of pregnancy is toxemia (eclampsia). It is generally related to excessive weight gain and high blood pressure. That is why you will notice that your blood pressure is taken at each prenatal visit to your healthcare provider. Even women without excessive weight gain may experience toxemia if their diet is not what's best for them. It's especially important to eat enough protein-containing foods that are low in fat. In addition, avoiding foods high in salt/sodium is important.

Keep your prenatal appointments so any early signs of eclampsia can be corrected promptly. Your healthcare provider will want to know about frequent headaches or unusual swelling. If you notice these things, be sure to contact your provider.

- **Prevents early birth by giving the baby the nourishment s/he needs daily.**

    I had the pre-eclampsia syndrome, real high blood pressure. Chen was born when I was 27 weeks pregnant. He weighed 1 pound, 9.5 ounces, and he stayed in the hospital for two months.

    Tao, 18 – Chen, 19 months

Your good eating habits help your baby grow and develop happily in your uterus until s/he is ready for life in your arms. Early birth is the cause of many physical and mental developmental delays. Also, babies that are smaller than average at birth often have difficulties with growth and development after they are born.

- **Helps with morning sickness and heartburn.**

    When I got pregnant, everything tasted nasty — for several months. But I got better toward the end.

    I live with my mom, and she helped a lot. She'd go buy the food I wanted and needed, and she tried to make sure I'd eat.

    Whitney, 17 - Mia, 2 weeks

If you eat from a variety of food groups you may be able to figure out which things help you avoid nausea and vomiting. Lukewarm liquids and crackers are a help, but so are frequent small meals that do not include fried or fatty foods.

For some women, eating a small meal at bedtime helps prevent that morning "feeling."

> *I get heartburn a lot. I've been keeping track of what might cause it and I just can't figure it out. I don't eat spicy foods or tomatoes. It seems that almost anything I eat gives me heartburn.*
>
> Nhu, 17 – almost 9 months pregnant

Eating frequent small meals, drinking fluids between meals, and avoiding greasy foods may help prevent heartburn. So can eating more fruits and vegetables. Don't lie down right after you eat. Take a walk instead.

• **Helps you feel less tired.**

The hormone shift of pregnancy is part of the cause of

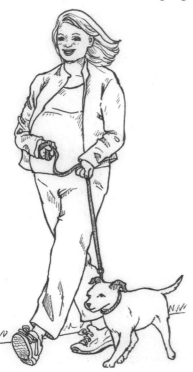

that early tiredness. As you begin to add the protein foods you need as well as a variety of fruits and vegetables, a lot of the sleepiness will fade away. Taking your prenatal vitamins, drinking plenty of water, and getting regular exercise will all improve your energy levels.

• **Makes you brighter and happier during your pregnancy.**

Just as baby's brain development will benefit from your good nutrition, so will yours. You may be surprised to find that you can pay attention longer when you have a balanced breakfast. Then you can recharge your body throughout the day with interesting choices from the many food groups.

"Okay," you say, "so what should I be eating while I'm pregnant?"

Follow This Guide

The U.S. Department of Agriculture recently replaced its Food Guide Pyramid with a pyramid made of a rainbow of colored, vertical stripes. The stripes represent the five food groups plus fats and oils. See pp. 49-50 for the **MyPyramid Food Guide** for adults.

At this time, MyPyramid has not been adapted for the special needs of pregnancy. Recommendations for foods to be eaten during pregnancy have not changed, however.

Food needs for pregnant teens and pregnant adults are somewhat different because the teen's body is still developing along with her baby. A pregnant teen needs all the good food an older pregnant woman needs *plus* an extra glass of milk.

Let's start with fats, oils, and sweets. Whatever your age, you need to eat very little of these — ration your greasy French fries and sugar-filled sodas. You need about 2600 calories each day while you're pregnant, only 400 more than before pregnancy.

Non-pregnant teens should consume about 46 grams of protein, 130 grams of carbohydrate, and 66 grams of fat daily. Now that you're pregnant, you need more protein, 50-70 grams (three servings), and more carbohydrate, 175 grams (four servings of vegetables, three of fruit, six of bread and cereals). But your need for fat remains the same, 66 grams.

Before pregnancy, I'd go out for fast food all the time. I ate as much greasy food as I wanted. I changed because I wanted my baby to be born healthy, and I

wanted to stay healthy. I didn't want to get too big.
I ate more fruits and vegetables than the greasy
foods while I was pregnant. I drank mostly water
rather than sweet drinks, no spicy food.

Gabrielle, 18 – Ambika, 15 months

First, Milk or Other Calcium-Rich Foods

While you're pregnant, if you're a teenager, you need
four or five servings from the milk, yogurt, and cheese
group. Do you drink low-fat or fat-free milk? If not, try it. If
you find you like the fat-free, you'll get about half as many
calories as with whole milk.

The healthiest cheese for a pregnant woman is low-fat
cottage cheese or ricotta cheese. Mozzarella cheese is somewhat lower in fat and sodium, but should be used moderately. This and all cheeses are higher than 30 percent fat unless
you buy the non-fat kind.

Spray can or glass jar cheeses are high in sodium and are
not a good choice for pregnant moms.

If you're lactose-intolerant, don't like milk, or for some
other reason aren't drinking milk, choose lactose-free
products such as soymilk and rice milk. Also eat other
things containing calcium such as foods and beverages
fortified with calcium and vitamin D.

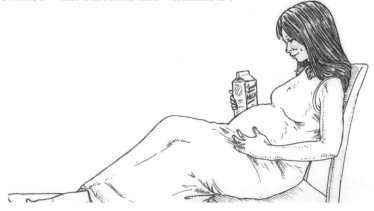

More Protein During Pregnancy

You and your fetus need significantly more protein than
you did before you got pregnant (a total of 50-70 grams, or
three servings). Meat, poultry, and fish provide a lot of protein. So do eggs, nuts, dried peas, lentils, and dried beans
like pinto and kidney beans. Peanut butter is another good
source of protein.

*When I got pregnant, I started eating a lot health-
ier and drinking more milk. I ate a lot of protein
because the doctor told me to.*

*We ate out a lot before I got pregnant, at least
twice a week. Then we stopped. Josh* (baby's father)
*helped a lot. Sometimes I'd want something, and he'd
say, "No, it's not good." He pretty much ate what I
ate. I don't like a lot of chicken or meat, but I ate it
anyway because I had to have the protein.*

Raquel, 19 – Giovanni, 4 months

When you eat meat or poultry, remove as much fat as
you can before cooking. Then bake, broil, or grill it.

Fish and shellfish are very good for you — but because
of the mercury content in many fish today, the FDA (Federal Drug Administration) suggests: Do not eat shark, swordfish, king mackerel, or tilefish because these fish contain
high levels of mercury. Limit yourself to about 12 ounces
(three average meals) weekly of such seafood as shrimp,
canned light tuna, salmon, tilapia, trout, herring, pollock,
and catfish. Salmon, trout, and herring are rich in omega 3
fatty acids, an important nutrient.

Recent research shows that fatty acids from the cold
water fish listed above are very important to brain development and childhood intelligence. Fish oil capsules avoid the
mercury problem and will provide benefit for both mother
and child. Fried foods should be strictly limited, as parts
of the hydrogenated fats sometimes used compete with the

desired fats.

If you have trouble eating enough meat to provide the protein you need, read chapter 8. It contains suggestions for vegetarians, people who choose not to eat meat. It is possible to get enough protein without meat, but it takes careful planning on your part. Eating plenty of protein foods helps prevent toxemia (eclampsia), as explained earlier.

Fruits and Veggies, Whole Grains

Now let's talk about fruits and vegetables. You need both because they are so rich in vitamins and minerals. Teens who eat a lot of fast foods often consume very few fruits or vegetables.

Before I got pregnant I ate anything and didn't worry about it – lots of fast foods. Me and my husband have been

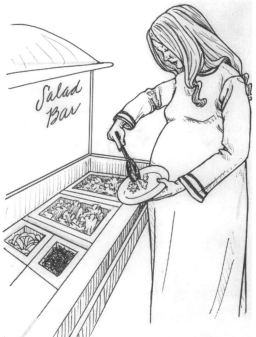

together for quite awhile, since I was 14. My husband is Puerto Rican so we eat a lot of rice and beans. He sees how eating right is good for us both. He grew up eating whatever.

While I was pregnant, of course I didn't eat deep fried foods. I ate a lot of seafood, a lot of vegetables, lots of carrots with the beta-carotene – I

only drank orange juice, water and milk.
While I was pregnant I craved a lot of things. I
craved Popeye's Chicken® but I never ate it because it
was deep-fried.

Vanesa, 19 – Andrea, 4; Josefina, 8 months

Fruits and vegetables are as good for you raw as cooked.
Salads with fruits and vegetables are healthy and provide
lots of important vitamins. Use dressings that are low in fat
and they will not make additional fat on your body.

Even if you don't like fruits and vegetables, try
them in a different way.
Put fruit in yogurt, try a fruit dip, or try apples in
caramel dip. It's not about you any more; it's about
your baby.

Chika, 16 - 4 months pregnant

For many teens, getting enough fruit is no problem. Eat a
banana with cereal for breakfast, take an apple to school for
a snack, and include fruit in your lunch. Already you have
your three portions.

Your fruit can be fresh or frozen, canned or dried. Limit
the fruit juice you drink because the juice is higher in sugar
and lower in other nutrients than is the whole fruit. Whole
fruit contains more fiber, too.

Consuming the needed four servings of vegetables is a
little harder for some people. Remember that you and your
baby will be healthier if you eat more dark green vegetables, broccoli and spinach, for example. Also especially
good for both of you are orange vegetables such as carrots
and sweet potatoes.

Growing up, I didn't like vegetables. Once I got
pregnant, I found different ways I could cook them. I
became more educated.

My grandmother — the only way she would cook broccoli was put it in the microwave. First I steam them, then add a little salt. They're still crunchy, and taste better.

Vanesa

You need six servings (one ounce each) of the bread, cereal, rice and pasta group each day. At least half of these foods need to be whole-grains, which means at least three ounces of whole-grain cereals, breads, crackers, rice or pasta every day.

One ounce is equal to one slice of bread, about a cup of breakfast cereal, or one-half cup of cooked rice, cereal, or pasta. For your additional portions of grains, the enriched kind is fine.

Your healthcare provider will probably prescribe prenatal vitamins for you. Even when you're absolutely sure you've eaten a good diet all day, you still need to take those vitamins. You may need an iron supplement, but check your vitamins first. Iron is probably included.

You also need to drink more water while you're pregnant, at least eight glasses (64 ounces) each day. This helps fight fatigue and prevent constipation. So does eating lots of fruits and vegetables.

So What's a Serving?

We talk a lot about servings. You need three servings of protein foods each day. Does this simply mean you need three servings, no matter how large or small the *portion?* Is a six-ounce steak one serving? (It's actually two.) Is a large hamburger bun one serving? It, too, provides two servings.

Servings as discussed here and in other food guides may not match the *portions* you eat. If you don't like peas, one tablespoon might be your *portion* while a *serving* of peas

and other vegetables means one-half cup. A serving of
lettuce salad means about a cup of salad.

Generally, the portions we're given, at least when we
eat out, are bigger than one serving. An order of spaghetti
might provide a two-cup portion. One-half cup of spaghetti
is a serving. Those two cups would actually provide four
servings from the grain group.

A serving of meat, two or three ounces, is about the size
of a deck of cards. Half a whole, small chicken breast is
one serving.

A large (4-ounce) bagel the diameter of a compact disk
provides four servings of grains. One-half of a 3-inch bagel
is one serving. A whole English muffin is two servings.

As you might expect, a medium apple, orange, or peach
equals one serving.

As you read labels, notice that sometimes the portion
for "one serving" is bigger than a serving as defined by the
MyPyramid guide.

Read the Labels!

As mentioned before, if you're a pregnant teen you need:
- 2600 calories
- 50-70 grams of protein
- 175 grams of carbohydrate
- 66 grams of fat

Most packages of food have charts showing information
about serving size and what is provided. Some even show
the percentage of calories from fat. For simple foods, such
as meats and fresh fruits and vegetables, you may have to
refer to another source such as a more detailed nutrition
book or the Internet.

One serving of fish or meat about the size of the palm of
your hand contains 20-25 grams of protein. A glass of milk
or one slice of cheese has about 9 grams.

For example, four glasses of milk and a good serving of fish or meat provides most of your protein for the day.

A piece of bread has 15-20 grams of carbohydrate, an orange, a nectarine or 12 grapes has 12 grams. Vegetables vary a lot. A tomato has 5 grams of carbohydrate and 21/2 stalks of celery have 4 grams, while most squash has 12, and a 3/4-pound potato has 25.

By contrast, the coating on a piece of fried fish or chicken has 25-50 grams of carbohydrate, and a short stack of pancakes with 1/4 cup of syrup has 105 grams. You can see why it's important to read the labels and the nutrition handouts at restaurants where you eat.

If you stick to the nutritious foods you and your baby need, and add very little food or drinks with high sugar content, your carbohydrate intake should not be a problem. See chapter 7 for more about sugar and other high-carbohydrate foods and drinks. See how easy it is to consume far too much carbohydrate if you drink sodas and eat foods with high processed sugar content.

The fats include things like butter, oil (both in dressing or in frying). Many fats are "hidden" in things like granola and packaged, processed foods. Lots of research shows that there is a relationship between too much fat in the diet and heart disease. In addition, too much fat stored on the body leads to diabetes and other serious diseases that no one wants. Too much fat eaten is stored as fat on your body.

Ask for the free nutrition handouts at your favorite fast food restaurants. Compare the cost in calories to the amount of food value. Think about that growing baby and your own growing body. Once you have identified the foods that are good for you, it will be easier to make good choices.

Learn to read the labels on food packages. Carefully check the macaroni and cheese label on p. 41, and study the information about labels on p. 40. Labels are important!

Reading Labels

1. Serving size. How many servings are in the package? How much will you eat? The label lists nutrient information for each serving size. If the label says a serving is one cup of macaroni, as this one does, then the serving actually provides two portions of grains.

2. Calories and **Calories from Fat.** You probably know that consuming too many calories makes us gain weight. We say a meal should seldom be more than 30 percent fat. But how do you know the percentage of fat? Divide the calories from fat by the total calories. According to this macaroni and cheese label, one serving provides 250 calories, and 110 are from fat. That means it is 44 percent fat.

3. Percent Daily Value (%DV). This tells you if the nutrients in a serving of this food provide a lot or a little of the total nutrients you need each day.

4. Fat, Cholesterol, and Sodium. Note the total grams of fat, cholesterol, and sodium. These are nutrients you need to limit, especially saturated fat, *trans* fat (very bad for you), and cholesterol. Also, it's best not to eat foods that contain more than 140 mg. of sodium per serving.

5. Energy and **Protein.** This section tells you the amount of carbohydrates — dietary fiber (good) and sugars (not good) — and protein the food contains. Dietary fiber helps with digestion and also helps prevent constipation. Your body uses protein to build lean body tissue mass — both for you and for your unborn baby.

6. Vitamins A and **C, Calcium, Iron.** You need lots of these. Look for foods that provide more than 30 percent of **%DV** of these vitamins and minerals.

Nutrition Facts

1 | Serving Size 1 cup (228g)
Servings Per Container 2

Amount Per Serving

2 | **Calories** 250   Calories from Fat 110

                   % Daily Value*

3 **Total Fat** 12g	**18%**
Saturated Fat 3g	**15%**
4 *Trans* Fat 3g	
Cholesterol 30mg	**10%**
Sodium 470mg	**20%**
Total Carbohydrate 31g	**10%**
5 Dietary Fiber 0g	**0%**
Sugars 5g	
Protein 5g	
6 Vitamin A	**4%**
Vitamin C	**2%**
Calcium	**20%**
Iron	**4%**

* Percent Daily Values are based on a 2,000 calorie diet. Your Daily Values may be higher or lower depending on your calorie needs.

		Calories:	2,000	2,500
Total Fat	Less than		65g	80g
Sat Fat	Less than		20g	25g
Cholesterol	Less than		300mg	300mg
Sodium	Less than		2,400mg	2,400mg
Total Carbohydrate			300g	375g
Dietary Fiber			25g	30g

Making Good Choices

So how do you make good food choices? For example, that taco salad with the pretty, fluted giant tortilla may seem like a good choice. It's a salad, it includes protein, and the tortilla is a grain. However, it has 870 calories (about 1/3 of your daily recommendation) and 50 percent of them come from fat.

At the same restaurant a choice of Burrito Supreme® – Chicken has only 410 calories of which 20 percent are fat. Each provides a healthy amount of protein. Add low-fat milk to the meal, and you have almost half the required protein that helps your baby's brain grow in the best way.

Make main dish selections that have 30 percent or less calories from fat and you probably won't need to worry about calories.

At first it may seem like a lot of trouble to figure all this out. But this information will help you for the rest of your life. It will also help you make decisions about what your child should eat to be healthy and strong.

In any case, learning to read labels and making good food choices will help you throughout life. *You will feel good and see your child develop well.*

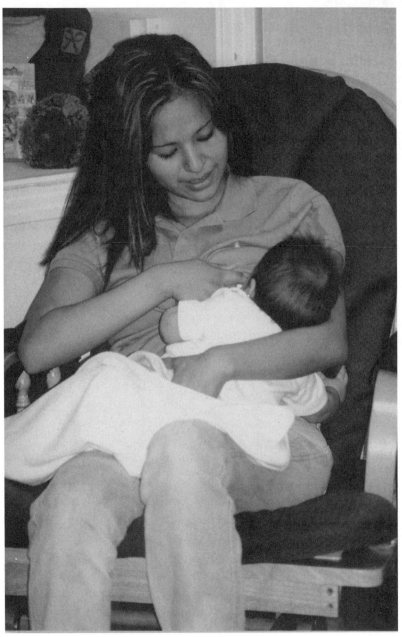

She's giving her baby the very best start.

2

Breast Is Best — for Baby and Mom

I breastfed him for two months, then bottle-fed. I highly recommend breastfeeding because you can notice right away when a baby is breast-fed, how healthy they look. You can just see right away.

Now I think if I ever have any more children, it will be breastfeeding for at least six months or a year.

Carlota, 18 – Luis, 4 1/2

I think the breastfeeding was the best thing I did. If I ever have another baby I will breastfeed because I know it has benefited both me and her

*. . . the bonding, knowing that you can help your child.
I think breastfeeding is good because they get the
antibodies from the mother which helps them. I have
noticed that the other babies in childcare who are
bottle-fed are sick a lot more.*

*It's also cost-effective. And when I first started, it
was easier to get the extra baby weight off.*

Kwanita, 17 – Noscha, 3 months

*I gave him some formula for awhile so I could have
somebody watch him for me so I could do my school-
work. This was about one bottle a day when he was a
month old, for two or three weeks.*

*Then I stopped doing that because I found I could
breastfeed while I studied. I got a Boppy® pillow and
could put that around my waist and sit cross-legged on
a chair. I could prop him there and type while
he nursed.*

Argentina, 18 – Danté, 6 months

A Gift for Your Baby

While you were pregnant, you were entirely responsible
for your baby's food. Ideally you, her mom, continue being
her complete food source for six months after she is born.
Breastmilk is the perfect food for babies. You'll be doing
your baby a big favor if you breastfeed throughout her first
year of life, longer if you wish.

You will be providing the best start for her by supplying a
natural defense against allergies and infections. Breast milk
contains fats needed for the best possible brain development
— she is likely to be smarter if you breastfeed. Breastfeeding also reduces the risk of obesity in your child, perhaps
even after she is grown. And you are likely to lose any extra
pregnancy fat sooner if you breastfeed.

*I breastfed for a whole year. It was cheaper, and
you lose weight faster. I never even thought of bottle-
feeding really. It was never like a choice.*

Hannah, 23 – Mackenzie, 41/2

Breastfed infants are less likely to get sick. They are less likely to suffer from diabetes, lymphoma, leukemia, Hodgkin's disease, and asthma, compared to children who were not breastfed. They are less likely to have diarrhea, ear infections, meningitis, and other infections. These are some of the reasons the American Academy of Pediatrics (AAP) recommends, with few exceptions, that all infants be breastfed at least during their first six months, and preferably for a year.

No wonder almost 3/4 of the children in the United States are breastfed for at least a short time. Two out of five are breastfed six months or more.

There are still other reasons to breastfeed. It's easier for you — no formula to mix or bottles to sterilize. You don't have to heat her milk. And when she's through nursing, no bottles to wash. Breastmilk is also much less expensive than formula. All you need to add to your good pregnancy diet are about 400 extra calories daily. An extra glass of milk and a sandwich is a good way to consume those extra calories.

Discussing Breastfeeding

*Since he turned four months old I started feeding
him rice cereal because I was so tired of everyone saying he wasn't getting enough nutrition – even though
he had plenty of wet diapers, he slept well, he gained
in weight – because none of them breastfed and they
would say such stupid things. I have to say, "You fed
your kids what you wanted and I feed mine the way
I want."*

Cynthia, 17 – Julian, 11 months

If you aren't considering breastfeeding, think of your reasons. Is it because of what other people say? You can explain the many advantages breastfeeding provides for your baby. You want to give your baby the best. Or you might even use Cynthia's comment, "You fed your kids what you wanted and I feed mine the way I want."

Or perhaps you're concerned breastfeeding might cause your breasts to sag. True, your breasts become larger during pregnancy, but wearing a good support bra during pregnancy and while you're breastfeeding helps prevent sagging.

Are you worried that baby's dad will feel left out if only you can feed your baby? Talk with him about how breastfeeding gives your baby (and his) the best possible start. Dad can still bathe baby, change his diaper, and love and cuddle him when he's not eating.

I know it's hard for girls my age and younger. I know some are afraid to breastfeed because they think breasts are sex objects and don't want a newborn baby hanging on it.

My aunt told me she felt that way, but when she started nursing her first baby she found it wasn't like that. It was a normal thing between the mother and her baby, very nurturing for both of them, good for bonding.

Lauren, 20 – Makayla, 15 months

Even if you don't want to breastfeed very long, consider this as a gift at least during your baby's first couple of weeks. At first your breasts won't make milk. Instead, they produce colostrum, a very nutritious yellowish substance which contains water, some sugar, minerals, and many important antibodies. These give your baby some protection against illness.

The "experts" say even a few drops of colostrum every

hour or so during those first couple of days is beneficial for
your baby. What amazing stuff!

*Why breastfeed? Because you're giving your kid
antibodies as long as you're breastfeeding, and it gives
you closeness to your baby. I have a relationship with
my baby. Julian knows I'm his mom. We have such a
close bond because of that. That's our time. He doesn't
look to anyone else to feed him.*

*When people say "I don't want to breastfeed," or
"It's gross," I try to explain, and say, "At least while
you're in the hospital, breastfeed — the colostrum is
so good for your baby."*

*I don't know why I hadn't thought about it before,
but during pregnancy I read up on breastfeeding. It's
so good for the baby. Why would your body create
something that's been around long enough so we know
it works? Sometimes now he has a bottle, but primarily
he breastfeeds.*

Cynthia

Those First Feedings

Do you know anyone else who is breastfeeding? When
you are beginning the wonderful task of feeding your baby,
talking with a mom experienced in the process can help.

*First days? Ooh, I was so discouraged like when
I was in the hospital my baby was real tired and he
would fall asleep. It would take ten minutes to wake
him up, and he would nurse only about five minutes,
and I got really really engorged. Then he couldn't latch
on because my nipple was so stretched out.*

*I was crying, and I was telling everyone that I'm
going to quit and put him on formula, but I didn't want
to. I had three nurses trying to help me get him to*

latch on.

Finally an older nurse got a nipple shield, and that worked. I was in the hospital 48 hours. I had to manually express milk because my breasts hurt real badly, they were really hard. He was crying. He never did have a bottle but he used his pacifier. I told them right away when I got to the hospital, "I'm breastfeeding."

Argentina

If you've never been around anyone who breastfed, you may wonder exactly how to start. First, the timing. Baby needs to nurse a few minutes within an hour of his birth. He does *not* need a bottle while he's in the hospital. Make sure everyone around you in the hospital knows you're planning to nurse, and that your baby is *not* to be given a bottle. This is very important.

Sometimes hospital personnel insist on providing that bottle. You can insist that they not. If you haven't delivered yet, prepare a brief birth plan detailing your wishes on anesthesia, people you want in the delivery room, etc. Include in big bold type, *"I will breastfeed my baby immediately after he is born. Do not give him a bottle!"*

Give a copy of your birth plan to your obstetrician, the hospital pediatrician, each nurse you see, and anyone else involved. If you tell them the American Academy of Pediatrics recommends no supplementary bottle, they will listen to you.

I was also strong about breastfeeding the first hour after he was born. I kept him in my room all the time I was in the hospital. I wanted to give myself time to get used to him.

Cynthia

Find out if your baby will be rooming with you in the hospital. This is the best plan for both you and your baby.

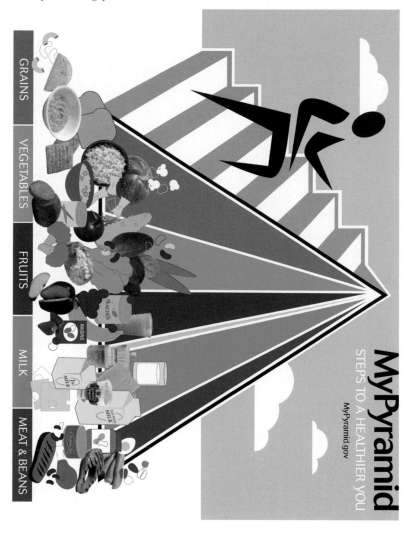

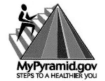

U.S. Department of Agriculture
Center for Nutrition Policy and Promotion
April 2005
CNPP-15

USDA is an equal opportunity provider and employer.

MyPyramid is your guide to healthy eating.

GRAINS Make half your grains whole	VEGETABLES Vary your veggies	FRUITS Focus on fruits	MILK Get your calcium-rich foods	MEAT & BEANS Go lean with protein
Eat at least 3 oz. of whole-grain cereals, breads, crackers, rice, or pasta every day	Eat more dark-green veggies like broccoli, spinach, and other dark leafy greens	Eat a variety of fruit	Go low-fat or fat-free when you choose milk, yogurt, and other milk products	Choose low-fat or lean meats and poultry
1 oz. is about 1 slice of bread, about 1 cup of breakfast cereal, or 1/2 cup of cooked rice, cereal, or pasta	Eat more orange vegetables like carrots and sweetpotatoes	Choose fresh, frozen, canned, or dried fruit	If you don't or can't consume milk, choose lactose-free products or other calcium sources such as fortified foods and beverages	Bake it, broil it, or grill it
	Eat more dry beans and peas like pinto beans, kidney beans, and lentils	Go easy on fruit juices		Vary your protein routine — choose more fish, beans, peas, nuts, and seeds

For a 2,000-calorie diet, you need the amounts below from each food group. To find the amounts that are right for you, go to MyPyramid.gov.

Eat 6 oz. every day	Eat 2 1/2 cups every day	Eat 2 cups every day	Get 3 cups every day; for kids aged 2 to 8, it's 2	Eat 5 1/2 oz. every day

Find your balance between food and physical activity

- Be sure to stay within your daily calorie needs.
- Be physically active for at least 30 minutes most days of the week.
- About 60 minutes a day of physical activity may be needed to prevent weight gain.
- For sustaining weight loss, at least 60 to 90 minutes a day of physical activity may be required.
- Children and teenagers should be physically active for 60 minutes every day, or most days.

Know the limits on fats, sugars, and salt (sodium)

- Make most of your fat sources from fish, nuts, and vegetable oils.
- Limit solid fats like butter, stick margarine, shortening, and lard, as well as foods that contain these.
- Check the Nutrition Facts label to keep saturated fats, trans fats, and sodium low.
- Choose food and beverages low in added sugars. Added sugars contribute calories with few, if any, nutrients.

Within an hour
after he's born,
put him to your
breast. Ask a
nurse to help you
place him on his
side, his tummy
against
yours.
Touch
baby's
lower lip
with your
finger or
nipple.
He'll
open
wide,

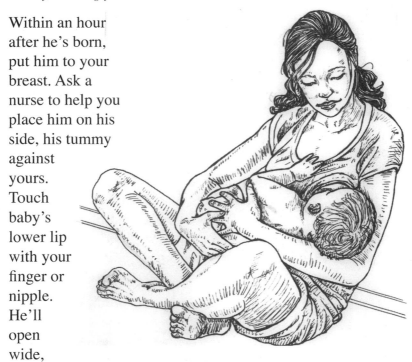

a rooting reflex action ready to go at birth. As his mouth
opens, bring him to your nipple.

Check to be sure his bottom lip curls out. If it doesn't,
pull down gently on his chin. Be sure he gets as much as
possible of the areola (dark area around the nipple) into his
mouth as he sucks. This is where the milk pools.

If he "latches on" properly, your nipples shouldn't get
sore. If it hurts, break the suction by putting your finger
between his mouth and your breast. Take him off, and latch
him on again with more of the areola in his mouth.

Nurse only two or three minutes on each side that first
time. He'll probably nurse 10-20 minutes on each side after
a week or two. Alternate the breast you offer first at each
feeding. In this way, he'll empty each one during every
other feeding.

Feed Her "On Demand"

The more often you nurse baby, the more milk you'll produce. Feed her "on demand," every time she wants to eat. She shouldn't have to cry to get a meal. Notice other signs she's hungry — increasing activity, rooting, mouthing. She needs to eat at least 8-12 times during each 24-hour period at first. Later on, you can probably work out a schedule that works for both of you.

When he first came home I fed him like constantly. They tell you that you will breastfeed more often, but nothing prepares you. It was every hour to 11/2 hours.
I wish more girls would stick with it, and know it gets easier, if they will just ride out the first hard days.

Caimile, 17 – Hajari, 4 months

Don't worry if your breasts are small. The amount of milk you make depends on how often your baby nurses. If your nipples are flat or inverted, you can wear breast shells inside your bra between feedings. These help bring out the nipples. A highly motivated baby will pull nipples out on her own.

The day after Julian was born a lactation consultant came in to the hospital and showed me how to get him to latch on and how to use the breast shield. I used the breast shield for three months. First to get him to latch on she used a syringe to show me there was something there. Then we tried the nipple shield.

Cynthia

Note: The nipple shield Cynthia mentions is made of soft plastic and is used if needed while baby nurses. It's very different from the nipple shell mentioned above. The shell is made of hard plastic and is used as needed between feedings.

Your nipples may get sore the first few days even if baby latches on properly. Expose your nipples to the air after each feeding and rub them with a little breastmilk.

It's best not to give your baby a bottle or pacifier at first. You can give her a better start at nursing if she doesn't get confused by sucking from a bottle or on a pacifier.

> *Perhaps I should have told them not to give Danté*
> *a binky right away. They took him to the nursery, and*
> *gave it to him. Then he didn't recognize my nipple.*
> *That made things harder. Danté shouldn't have had*
> *one until the breastfeeding was established.*
>
> Argentina

Note: According to recent research, a baby who, after the first couple of weeks, uses a pacifier when sleeping is less vulnerable to SIDS (Sudden Infant Death Syndrome).

How Much Is Enough?

How do you know when baby has enough milk? Whether he's breastfed or drinking formula, he will let you know. If he spits out the nipple (yours or the one on the bottle) and stops sucking, he's probably had enough. He may even fall asleep while he's eating. Don't insist that he suck longer (unless your baby has a special need that means he needs to be encouraged to suck). Let him be in control of his appetite.

Your baby is likely to grow especially fast when he's about two weeks old, again at six weeks, and at three months. At these times, he needs more food. You may think you don't have enough milk for him. You're probably right.

The solution is simply to nurse baby more often. That signals your breasts to make more milk. Your baby controls your supply of milk. Usually it takes about two days of nursing more often to make more milk. Then he will level out to nursing less often again. He'll also be more content.

You'll know he's getting enough milk if he has at least six wet and two dirty diapers each 24 hours, is gaining 4-7 ounces each week, and seems content for one or two hours between most feedings.

Don't think you need to hide away by yourself to nurse your baby. If you're out, throw a light blanket over baby while he nurses. Probably no one will even notice.

> *If I'm in the store and Julian needs to eat, I lift up my shirt and feed him. If people have a problem with it . . . To me, it's no different than feeding him a bottle.*
>
> Cynthia

Babies don't need additional water or any other food for the first four to six months, according to AAP.

While breastmilk is the healthiest food possible, the one nutrient missing is vitamin D, the sunshine vitamin. If you are breastfeeding only, or if your baby gets less than 16 ounces of formula a day, he needs a vitamin D supplement. Talk to your healthcare provider.

For more information about breastfeeding, see *Your Pregnancy and Newborn Journey* or *Nurturing Your Newborn* by Lindsay and Brunelli.

For personal help with breastfeeding, contact a lactation consultant. Ask your healthcare provider, or check with the hospital where you deliver. You could phone your local chapter of La Leche League (an organization of breastfeeding mothers). Or you could ask for help from WIC (Supplemental Feeding Program for Women, Infants and Children).

Your Diet

When you eat a variety of foods and breastfeed your baby, she will be able to "taste" these different flavors since they are transferred to your breastmilk. This means your baby learns about the foods you and your family enjoy. It also means she's more likely to accept new foods when she starts eating pureed food.

Occasionally a breastfed baby reacts to what her mom eats. If your breastfed baby cries or fusses more than usual, think about what you've been eating. You may want to quit eating a specific food for a couple of days. Is baby happier? Try eating that food again. Does it bother her? If so, you want to omit that food for awhile.

> *While breastfeeding, I ate basically the same things*
> *I ate while I was pregnant. I ate more calories because*
> *I needed to gain weight. I like milk so I drink quite a*
> *bit of milk. Breastfeeding is going real good. Abiba*
> *learned faster than Jabari did.*
>
> Abeni, 17 – Jabari, 16 months; Abiba, 6 weeks

To make breast milk, you need to have an adequate diet. Follow the same nutritious diet of vegetables, fruits, whole grain and protein foods, and dairy products (or another good source of calcium). As mentioned before, you need about 400 extra calories each day while you're breastfeeding. Most important — drink plenty of fluids, at least 12 cups of water, milk, fruit juice, and other non-sugary drinks daily.

Your healthcare provider will probably suggest you continue taking your prenatal vitamins if you're breastfeeding.

If you're vegan (you eat or drink no animal products, not even milk, cheese, or eggs), you're not getting enough Vitamin B_{12} in your food. It's important to have a reliable source of B_{12}, preferably from a supplement. This is necessary so your baby will get enough of this vitamin. Vitamin B_{12} is needed for the development of the nervous system and to prevent anemia.

Drugs/Smoking While Breastfeeding

Many medications are safe to take while you're breastfeeding, but check with your healthcare provider. Get

approval for any medication, even non-prescription items.
It's best to take the medication immediately after breastfeeding. Less of it will remain in your body for the next
nursing time.

If mom's milk has caffeine in it, baby's body can't get rid
of it easily. Limit your caffeine while you're breastfeeding.
One cup of coffee a day shouldn't harm baby. Too much
caffeine can make him nervous and irritable.

If you drink alcohol, it will pass through your milk to
your baby. It's best to abstain, but if you choose to drink, do
it immediately after you nurse. It's less likely to affect your
baby at his next feeding.

It's important that you not smoke while you're breastfeeding. If possible, you don't want anyone else to smoke around
your baby either. Second-hand smoke is dangerous to all
children, but especially to newborns. According to research,
it increases the risk of SIDS. It also increases your child's
chances of becoming asthmatic.

However, smoking is not a reason to forego breastfeeding. Even a mom who can't stop smoking should know that
her breastmilk is still the best food for her baby, according to
the Centers for Disease Control and Prevention. Of course it
would be better if she didn't smoke, or at least cut back on
the number of cigarettes. Her baby doesn't need the nicotine
but he does need her breastmilk.

Some birth control methods might interfere with your
milk production. Again, check with your healthcare provider.
You have plenty of good choices for birth control that will
not interfere with breastfeeding.

What About School or Work?

If you haven't finished high school, you know how
important it is for you to continue your education. If you're

working, it's probably because you need the money to support or help support your family. For working women, this generally means a 40-hour work week. For students, six-hour or longer school days are typical.

So how can you even consider breastfeeding your baby?

First, you'll probably have at least a month, preferably six weeks, at home after delivery. During this time, feed your baby often. This is the way to give breastfeeding a strong start. It's also an important part of bonding with your baby.

While you're home, think about possibilities for handling breastfeeding after you return to school or work. If you have a childcare center at school, you're lucky. If it's an alternative school (such as the one where we three worked), you shouldn't have a problem. You'll simply be called out of class to feed your baby whenever needed.

> *I'm going to breastfeed because of the nutrition benefits. The thing that got me was that all formula is not what breastmilk is, and I'm going to give my baby the real thing.*
>
> *The parenting program at school helps out a lot. At school you can pump once in the morning and once after lunch. Or you can go feed the baby. The childcare is two blocks away.*
>
> Chika, 16 - 4 months pregnant

If you're in a comprehensive high school with highly structured classes, it may be harder to feed your baby on demand — even if she is cared for on campus. Can you feed her at lunch time? Is there a mid-morning break?

Caimile's school had no provision for childcare, but she found a way to continue breastfeeding:

> *At WIC we met the peer workers, and I talked with a lactation consultant. We talked a lot before Hajari*

*was born and after. He doesn't take a bottle at all, and
I go to school for a full day.*

*So my mom brings Hajari to me during school so
I can nurse him at lunch. I go to lunch at 10:45 and
nurse him for 25 minutes. He's generally okay until I
get home at 2. I leave at 7:15 a.m. He nurses at night
every two hours.*

Caimile, 17 - Hajari, 4 months

Some babies, like Hajari, seem to "decide" that if Mom
isn't there much during the day, they'll make up for it by
nursing more often at night. If this happens to you, hopefully
you'll be able to go to sleep as soon as he finishes eating
(or sooner).

Teresa MacFarland, lactation specialist, has worked with
teen moms who choose to continue breastfeeding when they
return to school. She commented:

*I am completely convinced that it can be done, pro-
viding the teen mom has determination and an adult
advocate on her side. This may be the school nurse
or a faculty person (perhaps a breastfeeding mom as
well), or even her own mother.*

*I also know that some moms choose to stay on
independent study in order to breastfeed on demand.*

Pumping Works Too

Will you have no way to take your baby with you to
school or work, and no way to be with her during the day?
You can pump your breasts two or three times a day, put the
expressed milk in bottles, and refrigerate promptly.

Take the bottles home with you. (One friend always put
her car keys on the bottle of breastmilk in the refrigerator.
Then she wouldn't forget to take the milk home.) At least
one brand of pump has a section to hold an icepack to keep

the milk cold.

It's a good idea, if you're willing to get up really early, to pump your breasts before your baby wakes up. Your breasts make milk continuously, so you should still have enough for baby when she wakes up.

Your baby's caregiver will feed her the bottled breast milk the next day. If you ever have extra breastmilk, freeze it for use another day.

That extra bottle of breastmilk also gives Dad a chance to feed baby. Bonding between baby and Dad is important, too.

> *My work was good. When I went back to work, they were real cooperative about letting me take breaks. I had to pump, then bring it home.*
>
> Hannah, 23 - Mackenzie, 41/2

Find out about breast pumps. The good ones are expensive. So is formula. The cost of the formula you don't buy will pay for the breast pump before long. You may want to find one that pumps both breasts at once, a real time saver.

For more information, and perhaps the loan of a pump, talk with the WIC lactation specialist. Or call your local La Leche League. They might have a pump you could borrow. Or perhaps your school or workplace has or will buy one to be used by mothers who need it.

Where Will You Pump?

Of course you need a place to pump. If you're at school, can you go into the nurse's office? Or is there another place at school where you might find the privacy you need? Ask your counselor.

You may need to explain to the counselor why continuing breastfeeding is so important for your baby's development. Point out that your baby may be smarter when she starts school if you breastfeed her.

If you will be working at a job where pumping is possible, figure out where you will do it. In the ladies' lounge? An empty office? Or perhaps you work for a company that employs many young women of childbearing age. Do they provide a lactation center? Perhaps you could be the one that helps get such a center organized.

If you work for a fast food place, pumping probably wouldn't fit into your work schedule very well. How long are your work shifts? If you must work full-time, can you do this in three- or four-hour shifts, and feed your baby between shifts?

> *Breastfeeding was really hard in the beginning. I would give it to Ahmad, and sometimes he wouldn't take it, or sometimes my milk wouldn't come out. But I kept at it, and pretty soon it got easier.*
>
> *Now, when I go to work, I breastfeed him before I leave, and then when I get home, I breastfeed.*
>
> Latika, 18 - Ahmad, 3 months

If You Decide to Bottle-feed

> *I hold Nokomis when he takes the bottle. I didn't consider breastfeeding because we were going to give him up for adoption. My family hoped I would release. We changed our minds when he was born.*
>
> *Nokomis was in foster care for two weeks while we decided for sure. It's been good, really good since.*
>
> Kaliska, 16 – Nokomis, 9 months

If you choose to bottle-feed, copy the act of breast-feeding with skin-to-skin contact with your baby as you give her a bottle. You could push up your sleeve so baby feels your nice warm arm. Be sure to provide iron-fortified formula. Watch for her hunger cues. You don't want to wait until she's crying to feed her.

It's just as important to stop feeding her when she's had enough. "I'm full" cues might include lip smacking, slower sucking, and turning away from the bottle.

To make formula, simply follow the directions on the can.

> *I used powdered formula. You should add the warm water and then the formula – the formula gets all lumpy if you add it first.*
>
> Dolores, 18 – Enriko, 2 1/2 years

Never lay baby down and prop her bottle. She could choke, and she is more likely to get an ear infection if she drinks from a propped bottle. Most of all, she needs the love she feels from being close to you and cuddling in your arms while she drinks.

Your baby needs your breastmilk or formula throughout her whole first year. By six months, however, she will need other nutrients, especially iron and zinc. These minerals are essential for your baby's healthy physical growth and mental development. Zinc also helps baby maintain a healthy immune system.

So by six months you need to start feeding a little iron- and zinc-fortified cereal. She will also need fruits and vegetables high in vitamin C because this helps her body absorb the iron better. See the next chapter for information about introducing your little one to solid food.

Your child's attitude toward food now will influence how she feels about food throughout her life. *Your loving care is supremely important.*

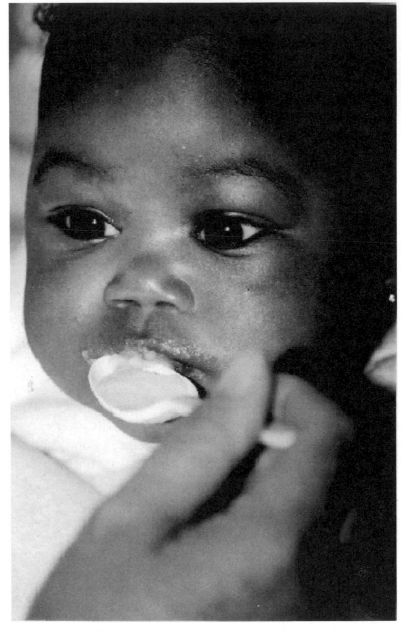

Eating solid food is serious business.
Now she can learn to enjoy a wide variety of tastes.

3

Strained, Smashed — Introducing Solid Foods

- **Breast Milk Is Still Important**
- **Baby Knows How Much**
- **His First Solid Food**
- **Preparing Baby's Food**
- **Freeze the Leftovers**
- **She Doesn't Like It?**
- **Keeping Your Baby Safe**
- **Eight Months — Time for Table Food**
- **Drinking from a Cup**
- **She's No Longer a Baby**

Moms and dads should be assertive in telling their family members not to give the baby cookies and other kinds of table food because they are just not ready for it. Just say, "Hey, this is my baby. We need to do things my way."
Argentina, 18 – Danté, 6 months

I don't give Julian much fried food because it doesn't do well with my stomach. I give him crackers but try to take the salt off. I don't give him French fries because someone told me that what I give him now will establish his eating habits for later on in life. I don't give him fries. I just think about all that grease.

Cynthia, 17 – Julian, 11 months

Breast Milk Is Still Important

Ideally, babies are completely breastfed their first six months. If he's bottle-fed, iron-fortified formula is all he needs until he's about six months old.

Your doctor may have recommended a vitamin D supplement when your baby was two months old, or even sooner. Baby needs to continue this until he is weaned to fortified whole milk at about one year. To get enough vitamin D from the milk, he needs to drink at least 17 ounces a day.

By his sixth month birthday, baby needs additional food. No longer does breast milk or formula contain all the other nutrients he needs. He is ready to learn to eat solid foods.

You have a fascinating challenge. This is the time your child's food habits and preferences start to develop. You want to encourage healthy eating habits right now.

I have learned not to say "Nasty" like, "Oh, that's nasty," like when you grind it up and it does look nasty. But if you say that, they will grow up thinking it's nasty.

Ameera, 17 – Aida, 12 months

Your feelings and beliefs about food and the way you feed your baby have a great deal to do with what he eats and how much. You and your baby can work together to develop the healthy eating habits you want for your child. With your help, he can develop a taste for a wide variety of the good foods he needs to grow well.

Baby Knows How Much

If Emma refuses to eat? I know that if she doesn't want to eat, I can't force her, so I just wait until she's ready. I could sit there and play games with her all day long and she might not eat anyway. She'll eat when she's ready.

Paige, 17 – Emma, 10 months

Did you know babies are born knowing how much food they need? Learn to read your infant's cues. When you're feeding her, tune in to her signals. When she's hungry, she may open her mouth and move toward the spoon you're offering her. She may try to swipe food toward her mouth. Or she may try to grab the spoon.

If she turns her head away or covers her face with her hands, she may be saying, "Enough already. I'm full." Offer her something to drink. If she still appears opposed to eating, it's time to stop.

Infants have very small stomachs. As a consequence, they need small, frequent meals. Start with only a teaspoon of food, and gradually give more. Always recognize signs that she's full.

Remember that her appetite one day may be quite different than it is another day. Some days she acts as if she's starving. Another day, she simply doesn't want to eat. Portions of food you give her will vary to meet her needs.

If she doesn't want to eat, I figure she's not hungry. I wrap it up and put it in the fridge, then heat it up for her later. Then there are times when she's really hungry, and has two bowls of cereal and I think, "Holy cow, girl!" I don't try to limit her food, nor do we force her to eat. I will never say, "You don't leave the table until you finish your food." If you're full, you're full.

Ameera

Never insist that she finish the amount you selected for her. Always cleaning one's plate is not necessarily a good thing, no matter what your grandma may say.

You decide what foods to offer your child and when to offer them. Then let your child decide whether and how much to eat. This is how you teach your child to respect her appetite. If she's hungry, she will eat heartily. When she's full, she will stop. This is how she learns to regulate her own food intake.

A lot of obese adults never learned this simple practice. Too many of us eat whatever is in front of us, providing we like the food. A child who has not been pushed into eating can be a good example for the rest of us.

His First Solid Food

So your baby is about six months old. He can sit up with some support, and seems ready for a little solid food.

Start with iron-enriched rice cereal, the kind for babies that you buy in a box. Mix about a teaspoon of cereal with three or four teaspoons of breast milk or formula. You'll have a very thin mixture.

Put him in an infant seat or on your lap. Use a long-handled spoon with a small bowl that fits easily in his mouth. (Feeding him with a regular teaspoon would feel to him like you'd feel eating with a big serving spoon.) Bring the spoonful of cereal to his lips, but don't try to put it in his mouth.

At first he will use his sucking skills to get the cereal in his mouth. Offer him a couple of spoonfuls. If he doesn't want it, wait a few days, then try again. Gradually make the cereal a little thicker.

He will like his food served at room temperature. There's no need to make it hotter.

I started giving her cereal about three weeks ago,
and I give it to her once a day. Now she eats every
three hours including nighttime. She wakes herself up

like "I'm starving," and she may do that until she's
15 pounds. I'm exhausted. My mom doesn't help me
during the nighttime because she has to go to work.
Monique, 18 – Ashley, 5 months

Not long after you start offering a little rice cereal, slowly start feeding him a little strained vegetables and fruits. Starting with vegetables means he won't get used to only the sweet taste of fruit.

Always wait three or four days before you offer a different food. Then if baby shows an allergic reaction, such as a slight rash or upset stomach, you'll know which food probably caused the problem.

As a starter, mash part of a banana and offer it to him. Cover the remaining part with some plastic wrap and put it in the refrigerator. You don't need to buy a jar of strained banana. It's very easy to fix yourself.

Go on to applesauce, mashed carrots, squash, sweet potatoes, pears, and peaches. Mashed ripe avocado is also a good choice. He will probably start with a teaspoon of fruit or vegetable, increasing to 1/4 to 1/2 cup daily given in two

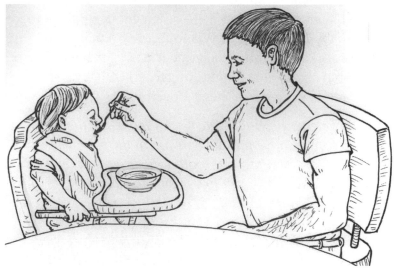

or three feedings.

If you buy the Stage 1 strained baby food, choose those
that have only one ingredient. Skip the desserts and
the mixtures.

Preparing Baby's Food

*Pancho had baby food from about five or six
months until about a month ago when he didn't really
want anything to do with the baby stuff.*

*He wants the table food. He loves spaghetti. We
aren't going to give him a hot dog or something real
spicy. When we have chicken, we cook twice what he
will eat and I save part for the next night in case we
have something spicy.*

Querida,18 – Pancho, 10 months

You don't have to buy the jars of baby food. You can
mix it quite easily by yourself if you have a blender. You
can press the food through a sieve or you can buy an inexpensive baby food grinder. You'll probably find the grinder
easier for preparing small amounts of food for your baby.

The blender will be handy if you fix enough pureed food
to feed baby now with leftovers to freeze. Actually, the
blender works better than the grinder during that short time,
from about six to eight months of age, when baby needs
very smooth, strained, or Stage 1 baby food.

*Josie eats vegetable crackers. I make her food.
Whatever we have for dinner, I put in the blender and
she eats it. If we have broccoli, I don't put salt on it, of
course. I don't add stuff like if I make mashed
potatoes, I don't add salt.*

*I started at five or six months. I prepared every-
thing except the rice cereal. She doesn't like peaches.
She loves sweet potatoes. I cut them up in squares and*

pop them in the oven. I don't put anything on them. If they want a little salt or sugar, they can add it.
Vanesa, 19 – Andrea, 4; Josephina, 8 months

Steaming food is better for baby (and the rest of us) than boiling it. Food cooked in boiling water loses valuable vitamins and minerals. To steam, you need an inexpensive steaming basket to insert in your cooking pot. It holds the food above the boiling water as it cooks.

Steam cut-up vegetables over boiling water in a covered pan until tender. Then mash or blend them. You may need to add a little cooking water to get the right consistency.

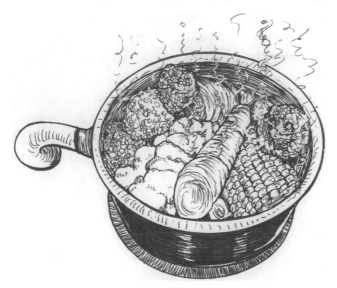

You could also use vegetables canned in water without seasonings for baby. Blend or grind up.

When you're cooking for your family, take baby's portion out before you add salt, sugar, and other seasonings. Babies like bland foods. A craving for salt happens from eating salted food. You're fixing food for your baby, not you, so don't season it. You want it to taste good to her, even if you find the taste too bland.

Emma was about five or six months when we started giving her the baby cereal and the jars of baby food. Now everything we eat we fix for her. If we have a roast, potatoes, carrots, we put it in the blender, all together. She really likes it. We still buy some jars of food so she will have what she needs.

Paige, 17 – Emma, 10 months

We all need at least five servings of vegetables and fruits each day — even babies. But how much is a serving? When she first starts eating fruits and vegetables, it may be as little as one teaspoon or even less. For older babies, a reasonable serving is about 1/4 cup or 1/2 container of pureed food.

If you prepare most of baby's fruits, vegetables and meats yourself, you'll save quite a lot of money. You can do it fairly quickly.

You can cook fruit for baby — apples, peaches, pears, plums, apricots. Wash, peel and cut the fruit into small pieces and remove the pits. Steam until tender, 10-20 minutes. Do not add sugar. Blend until smooth with a baby food grinder or blender.

If he's at least six months old, you can fix some uncooked fruit for baby. Wash and peel an apple, pear, peach, or apricot. Add a little water, and blend.

Fruit canned in water or its own juices (no sugar added) can also be blended or ground up for baby.

When you cook meat for your family, blend it until it's smooth. Add a little water or broth as needed.

Freeze the Leftovers

To freeze leftover baby food you've prepared, put the food in molded ice cube containers. When it's frozen, use freezer bags for storing. Keep meat, vegetable and fruit cubes separate.

When you're ready to use them, warm the food cubes over boiling water or in a small egg-poaching pan. Remember, warming just to room temperature is fine with baby.

If you're going out to eat and you're taking your baby, put the frozen food cubes in a little dish and take it along. The food will probably be thawed by the time you get to the restaurant.

Each time you cook a vegetable for your family, cook extra and freeze. This makes it much easier to offer baby a variety of tastes, no matter what the family eats.

She Doesn't Like It?

I used to hear, "You can't get down from the table until you eat," but I think I don't eat what I don't like and why should he? And I don't eat when I'm full, so Julian shouldn't have to either. There's a point when he needs to eat, but if he's eating well enough, why force him to the table and try to get him to eat?

Cynthia

Your little one may tell you she doesn't like a new food by spitting it back out as fast as you feed her. Or she may simply keep her mouth shut and turn her head away when she sees something new being offered. Many babies tend to be leery of new foods.

If your baby rejects a new food, perhaps mashed sweet potatoes, don't assume she will never have the health benefits that come with eating sweet potatoes. Wait a few days, then offer her sweet potatoes again. She still refuses? Try again another day. Sometimes it takes ten, even 15 times of seeing and perhaps trying a tiny bite of a new food before baby will accept it.

Your goal is for your child to enjoy a wide variety of healthy foods. Patiently offering many different foods is worth the effort. If she learns to eat new foods when she's tiny, she's more likely to accept a wide variety of foods when she's older.

Even if she doesn't appreciate the specific food you offer, you need to be patient and pleasant. If mealtime is an enjoyable time, she's more likely to try new foods.

By seven or eight months, she will enjoy picking up pieces of food with her fingers and eating them. She'll like such foods as soft cheese, unsalted crackers, small pieces of tortilla, tofu, and toasted whole grain bread. Avoid breads with nuts or large seeds. She may be more likely to accept spoonfuls of the food you're giving her if she can also pick up bits of food to put in her mouth by herself.

Keeping Your Baby Safe

If you buy the jars of baby food, don't feed your baby directly from the container. Take out the amount you think he'll eat and put it in a dish. If he doesn't eat all of that portion, throw out the rest of it. Do not save it to give to him later. This is not safe.

After you open the jar of food, put the unused portion into the refrigerator immediately. It will stay fresh and safe for one or two days. Write on the lid the date you opened it.

Fish is good for baby — but do not offer shark, swordfish or other large predatory fish because of the mercury content.

Follow the three "S" rules when you feed your baby: While he's eating, keep him *safe, seated,* and *supervised.* Don't let him eat while he's playing. He should be in his high chair, your lap, or a safe chair when he eats *or drinks.* It's safer, and he's developing good eating habits.

You need always to be with him when he's eating or drinking. During these early months, he could gag on a food because he's moving from pureed to lumpy food. He may also gag when he eats too fast or puts too much food into his

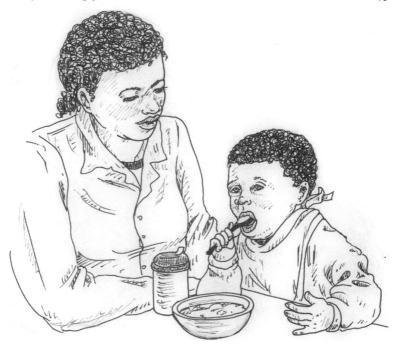

mouth. You need to be there.

*The main thing that kind of scares me is making
sure it's small enough for Pancho to eat it without
choking. We both know how to do CPR on him.*

Querida

Don't ever put cereal or other foods in his bottle. He
sucks on his bottle, but he needs to eat solid food. Putting it
in the bottle is also dangerous because he could choke.

Don't give your baby honey until he's at least a year old.
It can cause infant botulism (food poisoning).

Eight Months – Time for Table Food

*Our eating habits are healthy, we don't eat out, and
Pancho loves the table food much more than the baby
food. We just chop the meat up real fine.*

Querida

By the time she is eight months old, she may want between three and nine tablespoons of cereal daily, spread out in two or three feedings. After making sure she's not allergic to rice cereal, try barley, then oats. Always wait several days between offering each new food.

> *I always make sure I do it step by step – barley cereal is the only thing Aida can't eat. She would throw it up but she eats other cereals, rice, oatmeal. With the rice I mash up some banana and put it in the cereal and she loves that.*
>
> Ameera

Most babies need truly smooth food only until they're about eight months old. By this time, you can chop and mash table foods for her.

By eight to ten months, she can handle small amounts of pureed meats and poultry. She can also get her protein from egg yolk that you have boiled and cut into small pieces she can feed herself.

Well-cooked and mashed beans with soft skins such as lentils, split peas, pintos, and black beans are good sources of protein. So is tofu. If you feed your baby tofu, just mash it first. If you are vegetarian, and you plan not to serve meat to your child, you need to serve her plenty of these other protein foods.

Two to four tablespoons of protein food per day is enough at this age.

Offer her more finger foods such as small pieces of ripe banana, unsweetened Cheerios®, and teething crackers. She can also eat well-cooked spiral pasta. Lightly toast bagels, then cut them up into little pieces and offer her some.

Try offering scrambled eggs. Some days she'll like feeding herself. Other times, she'll appreciate your help.

You can also start offering her apple or pear juice. She

shouldn't have orange or other citrus juice until she's at least a year old. This is because some babies are allergic to citrus fruits their first year.

Limit the apple or pear juice to 1/4 cup a day because of its sugar content. Dilute the juice with an equal amount of water before serving it to her. This will taste good and provide only half as much sugar as straight juice.

Are you eating out occasionally? She'll probably eat a little of your hamburger and bun. Add a jar of Stage 2 or 3 fruits or vegetables plus her formula, and she'll have a balanced meal. Or take the frozen cubes of fruits or vegetables you prepared instead of the more expensive Stage 2 or 3 jars. She's likely to prefer the taste of her home-cooked food.

This is a messy time for your baby — and for you. While she's learning to feed herself, food is likely to end up on the floor, be smeared in her hair, and on her face. Some will go in her mouth. This is the way she learns.

Just put a thick layer of newspapers under her chair. When she's through eating, roll up the newspapers and throw them out or compost them. It's an easy way to handle her mess.

Drinking from a Cup

By the time baby is seven or eight months old, start teaching him how to drink water from a small cup. A "training" cup with a spout helps him adjust from sucking milk to being able to drink from a cup. He's also less likely to dump formula or water from a training cup than a regular cup.

Babies and toddlers need breast milk or formula, water, or a little unsweetened fruit juice in their cup. They seldom need anything else. Soda, coffee, tea, or fruit drinks should not be given to him at this stage. He should not have the sugar and/or caffeine they contain.

You may decide to continue breastfeeding after he's a year old. Serve other liquids to him in a cup.

The end of the first year is a good time to wean a bottle-fed baby from the bottle to the cup. Unless he's allergic to milk, he needs to become accustomed to drinking *whole* milk (not low- or non-fat). Offer four ounces in a cup, four times a day with meals or snacks. He should not drink more than 24 ounces each day. Otherwise he might not have an appetite for the other foods he needs.

If your child does have an allergy to milk, check with your doctor for the best milk substitute for him.

She's No Longer a Baby

Now he eats everything basically. I don't give him hard stuff he can choke on – or corn or honey. My grandma cooks things extremely well done. Usually I just take little pieces that I know he can't choke on.

Cynthia

By ten months she is no longer an infant. Not only does she pick up food and put it in her mouth, she's also trying to use the spoon herself. You can start offering yogurt and mashed cottage cheese, even soft pasteurized cheese. She may want as much as 1/3 cup of yogurt or cottage cheese, perhaps 1/2 ounce of cheese.

Continue giving her iron-fortified cereals. By now, if she shows no symptoms of allergy caused by rice, barley, wheat, or oat cereal, you can add mixed cereal to her diet.

Her fruit can be cut into cubes or strips or mashed. She can handle bite-size soft cooked vegetables such as peas (with the skin broken) and carrots. She's even ready for a small serving of combination foods such as macaroni and cheese and casseroles.

She likes table food – macaroni and cheese, mashed potatoes, peas, very thin pieces of meat like ham and turkey, real little pieces.

She likes vegetables. I think her favorite is broccoli and cheese. I make them and put them in a food processor and blend it.

I put spaghetti, Salisbury steak and rice together and blend it for her. I add a little formula so it won't be so thick. She likes to eat it herself.

Ameera

Continue to introduce new foods one at a time with at least three days wait before trying another new item. If you notice she has a rash or an upset stomach after a particular food, discontinue that food for a while.

Now she needs three or four meals per day plus snacks. Meals and snacks need to be planned to meet her nutrition needs. She does not need sweets or fried foods, and she should have little or none of either. (See chapter 7.)

Now you can start including your baby in family meals. She will enjoy being sociable as she eats.

I usually eat with the family, and I feed Emma while we're eating. If there's an argument, she wants to be right there. We eat around the table. It's easier than trying to haul her in the other room and do everything in front of the TV. And she likes sitting there and talking with the family. She really can't talk but has her own little conversations.

Paige

Continue offering your baby a wide variety of foods. Let mealtime be a happy time. She probably won't eat everything you want her to eat all the time, but she will develop good eating habits under your patient guidance.

Teaching her to eat the healthy foods she needs is a great gift for your child.

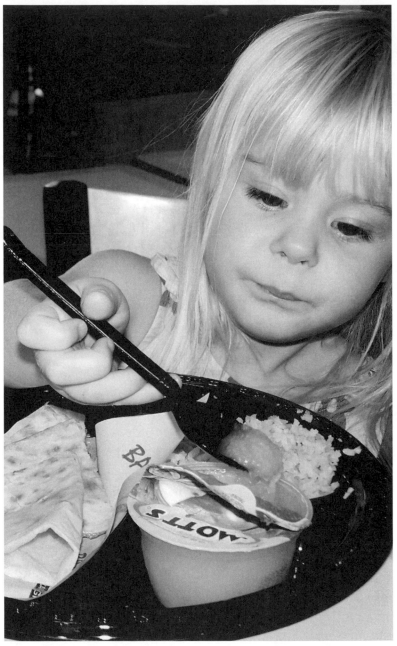

Her fast foods are a nutritious quesadilla, applesauce, and milk.

4

Fast Food
and Healthy Eating

Obesity is such a big factor here in the U.S. because fast food is so accessible. It's everywhere. They advertise so much to the kids, and then the kids whine and whine. Finally the parents give in, and they shouldn't. It's too easy — "Let's just go to McDonald's® and I won't cook today." I think that's why we have such a problem, because we're lazy.

When I work all day, I don't want to cook when I get home. It's hard with both parents working, and neither one wants to cook.

Caimile, 17 – Hajari, 4 months

Normally at fast food places, Mackenzie orders the chicken happy meal with a salad which strikes me as odd, but that's her choice. She doesn't drink the soda there. She gets the chocolate milk.

Hannah, 23 – Mackenzie, 41/2

When I got pregnant, I started eating less junk food. Before pregnancy, we were going out at least three times a week for fast foods. We changed to about once every two weeks or so.

Ameera, 17 – Aida, 12 months

Fast Foods Everywhere

Fast foods are around us everywhere – in schools, at malls, in every neighborhood, at the movies, and in the grocery store. They are popular with many people because of their convenience, price, and attractiveness, especially to children. Children are also attracted to them because of advertising on TV and the cute bags with toys in them.

We decided this fast food chapter needed to come before the chapters on feeding toddlers and preschoolers. This is because so many babies and toddlers are given "just a taste" of French fries, for example, when they are very young. Then they quickly develop a taste for them.

In fact, French fries are one of the three most common vegetables eaten by babies 9-10 months old. By 15-18 months, they eat more French fries than any other vegetable. Greasy French fries are a very poor substitute for nutritious vegetables.

We aren't telling you all fast food is bad. We are suggesting you make good choices when you do eat fast foods. Also remember that your baby doesn't have to try everything you eat. Your modeling of good eating is very important. But if you're eating French fries, try offering your baby a cracker instead. Otherwise, you're *teaching* him to like the fat and salt in the French fries. If he doesn't develop this taste now, he'll be healthier. *It's up to you.*

I think kids are overweight because their parents eat a lot of snacks. They should cut down on snacks, candy, and fast foods. That's why I try to stay away from it.

I give Jabari crackers, like graham crackers for his snack instead of a bunch of candy. A lot of people are overweight because their parents give them whatever they want to eat.
Abeni, 17 – Jabari, 16 months; Abiba, 6 weeks

As you plan healthy food choices for yourself and your child, are you including trips out for fast foods? It *is* possible to find nutritious foods at some of the fast food restaurants. Know that it is extremely important to make the best possible choices, however, if you're eating fast foods.

There are good, okay and poor offerings, both at eating-out locations and in the grocery store. Pick up the nutrition charts at your favorite restaurants. Then let's look at some of them and make comparisons. These will help you reach your goal of healthy family eating.

Facts to Remember
Teens 14-18 years old should be eating
- about 2200 calories each day
- 46 grams of protein
- 130 grams of carbohydrate
- 66 grams of fat

Pregnant teens need
- 2600 calories each day
- 50-70 grams of protein
- 175 grams of carbohydrate
- 66 grams of fat

Breastfeeding mothers should have
- about 3000 calories per day
- 60-70 grams of protein
- 210 grams of carbohydrate
- 78 grams of fat

Children under six months need all of their calories to come from breastmilk or formula. You'll be introducing other foods at the end of that period, mostly for the purpose of introducing solid food eating style and taste. Cereal provides iron and zinc that infants need by six months.

Children from six to 12 months still need their breastmilk or formula as their main source of nutrition. Toward the end of her first year, your baby may be eating 21/2 containers of baby food or 11/4 cups of home-prepared food each day.

Toddlers from one to three years old need
- 1500 calories each day
- 13 grams of protein
- 130 grams of carbohydrate
- 35 grams of fat

Children from four to eight need
- 1700 calories each day
- 19 grams of protein
- 130 grams of carbohydrate
- 47 grams of fat

Watch Out for Sodium in Foods

In addition to the sugars and fats in fast food and prepared foods, another enemy of good health is sodium. Keeping sodium low in the diet is important for everyone.

This becomes a really big issue during pregnancy. Too much sodium in the diet contributes to high blood pressure and toxemia/eclampsia, a very serious condition.

> *One thing I noticed is when there was too much*
> *salt in my food, I would swell up. I had to limit the salt*
> *because I would swell up pretty bad.*
>
>   Nhu, 17 - almost 9 months pregnant

Throughout life high blood pressure is an important health issue for many families. Learning now about how to use less sodium-containing foods, especially salt, is important.

The recommended amount of sodium intake per day, according to the National Institute of Health, is 1500-2400 mgs/day for adults. One teaspoon of salt contains 2300 mgs (milligrams) of sodium. *Read* labels, and add little or no salt to foods you prepare. Use spices, salsa, and other seasonings to season foods whenever possible and add no salt.

Even egg dishes, which many people salt heavily, taste good with salsa, or with low sodium cheese (such as swiss cheese) on them. Or how about adding pepper only? There are also salt substitutes available in the market. Ask your health care provider if that's what they recommend.

Children should have only about 1000-1500 mgs/day of sodium. By offering the smaller amounts of food they prefer, they also get less salt.

The information on pp. 81-82 is important. It helps you know when you and your child have had enough of each food type for the day. Most of the calories that are good for children come from fruits, vegetables, milk, protein foods, and grain products (bread, cereal, crackers). No total meal choice should be higher than 30 percent fat.

Best Fast Food Choices

> *It's hard, especially now with the pregnancy crav-*
> *ings. I'm tempted to eat at McDonald's® or go get*
> *pizza and fries. Sometimes I give in. But we seldom*

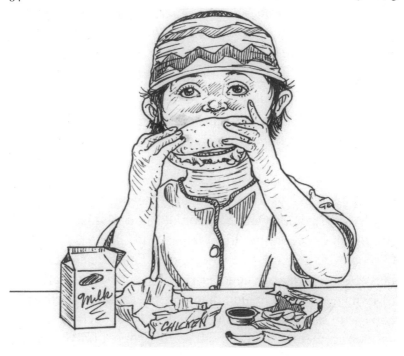

*eat fast food because my doctor said I shouldn't eat
greasy foods, and to cut back on fast foods.*
                Katrina, 18 – 7 months pregnant; Salvador, 19 months

Katrina is wise to avoid fast food most of the time. But
when she "gives in," she may find it possible to order foods
that provide the nutrients she needs. Several of the fast food
restaurants now offer some healthy choices. You don't *have*
to order a double-burger with bacon and cheese, large order
of fries, and a giant soda with the following nutrients:

	Calories	Protein	Carbs	Fat	Sodium
Double burger					
w/bacon, cheese	730	47	46	40	1720
Fries - large order	570	6	70	30	330
Giant soda	310	0	86	0	20
Totals	**1610**	**53**	**202**	**70**	**2070**

Wow! That's *more* protein, carbs, and fat and almost as much salt and calories as you need for your *entire day*!

Now let's look at some more reasonable choices. For Mom, these are based on 550 calories for each of three meals. This leaves an additional 550 calories for snacks. **Note:** Protein, carbohydrate, and fat are measured in grams, while sodium (salt) is listed in milligrams.

Good Choices for Mom

	Calories	Protein	Carbs	Fat	Sodium
Grilled steak taco fresco style	280	12	21	5	650
Pintos and cheese	180	10	20	7	700
Ice water with fresh lemon	0	0	0	0	0
Totals	**460**	**22**	**41**	**12**	**1350**

Ask for pintos without cheese to lower the fat and sodium in your meal.
(Taco Bell®)

	Calories	Protein	Carbs	Fat	Sodium
1 slice (14 in.) cheese pizza	220	11	25	8	610
1 slice (14 in.) veggie lover pizza	190	9	26	6	570
Water (Drinking water means more pizza!)	0	0	0	0	0
Totals	**410**	**20**	**51**	**14**	**1180**

Pizza Hut®

	Calories	Protein	Carbs	Fat	Sodium
Grilled chicken breast without skin	153	29	0		540
Garden salad	111	5	8		271
2 corn tortillas	140	9	30		60
Iced tea without sugar	0	0	0		10
Totals	**404**	**43**	**38**		**881**

(El Pollo Loco®)

	Calories	Protein	Carbs	Fat	Sodium
Bacon ranch salad with chicken					
WITHOUT the bacon	247	29	12	3	749
Vinaigrette dressing	40	0	4	3	440
Low fat milk	100	8	12	2.5	125
Totals	**387**	**37**	**28**	**8.5**	**1314**
(McDonald's®)					
Chicken McNuggets (6)	250	15	15	15	450
Side salad, vinaigrette dressing	40	0	4	3	440
Low fat milk	100	8	12	2.5	125
Totals	**390**	**23**	**31**	**20.5**	**1015**
(McDonald's®)					
Regular roast beef sandwich	320	21	34	14	953
Low fat milk	100	8	12	2.5	125
Totals	**420**	**29**	**46**	**16.5**	**1078**
(Arby's®)					

If you're determined enough to take off the chicken skin and breading and ask for mashed potatoes with no gravy, and don't put butter or salt on your corn, the following menu would be fine:

	Calories	Protein	Carbs	Fat	Sodium
Chicken breast *without skin or breading*	140	29	0	3	410
Mashed potatoes *without gravy*	110	2	17	4	320
Corn on cob (3 inches) *no salt or butter*	70	2	13	1.5	15
Ice water with fresh lemon	0	0	0	0	0
Totals	**320**	**33**	**30**	**8.5**	**745**
(KFC®)					

Fast Food Breakfast

	Calories	Protein	Carbs	Fat	Sodium
Egg McMuffin®	300	17	30	12	860
Low fat milk	100	8	12	2.5	125
Orange juice	140	2	33	0	5
Totals	**540**	**27**	**75**	**14.5**	**990**

(McDonald's®)

	Calories	Protein	Carbs	Fat	Sodium
Sourdough egg and cheese	392	17	40	12	1058
Orange juice	140	2	33	0	5
Totals	**532**	**19**	**73**	**12**	**1063**

(Arby's®)

Although these meals contain a nice supply of protein, you need to plan your remaining meals carefully. You'll need to drink more milk or consume other dairy products.

These meals contain only one serving of either a fruit *or* vegetable, and some have none. You need at least five. (One-half cup is a serving of vegetables.) You'll also need several additional one-ounce servings of whole grains. If you're pregnant or breastfeeding, you'll need additional protein, too.

Eating more than one fast-food meal per day will most likely mean a day high in sodium intake. Eating that much salt over time, especially during pregnancy, contributes to increased swelling, higher blood pressure, and possibly toxemia (eclampsia).

Fast Food for Toddlers

	Calories	Protein	Carbs	Fat	Sodium
1/2 small hamburger	130	6.5	16	4.5	215
Low fat milk	100	8	12	2.5	125
Apple Dippers	105	0	23	1	40
Totals	**335**	**14.5**	**51**	**8**	**380**

(McDonald's®)

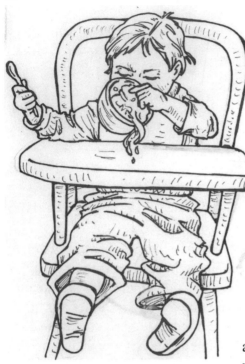

This morning Savannah had potatoes with an egg. In the middle of the day we ate at McDonald's — French fries, one hamburger and juice. We shared.

Tonight she will have meat with vegetables.

Lareina, 17 - Savannah, 2½

Breakfast out for a toddler needs to be unsugared cereal from home. Buy low-fat milk to add to the cereal.

You could add orange juice at 140 calories, 2 grams protein, 33 carbohydrates and 0 fat for him too. Apple dippers without sauce can be ordered at breakfast if available. Add 35 calories and eight carbs.

He will need a good supply of fruits and vegetables, whole grains, and milk in his remaining meals and snacks.

Hamburger for Preschoolers

Kendall likes McDonald's® because she likes the Happy Meal. She loves fries.

We try not to eat out as much as we used to. The doctor said too much fast food was bad for Kendall because of the obesity problem. She's never been overweight, but he said this could become an eating habit.

So we changed. We used to eat out about four times a week. Now Sunday is family day and we eat out. That's all.

Ukari, 19 – Kendall, 3

	Calories	Protein	Carbs	Fat	Sodium
Small hamburger	260	13	33	9	430
Low fat milk	100	8	12	2.5	125
Fruit cup (apples and grapes)	24	0	9	2	0
Totals	**384**	**21**	**54**	**13.5**	**555**

Just as with the toddler menu, this gives a preschooler enough protein. He will need more fruit, vegetables, milk, and whole grains in his other meals and snacks.

Breakfast out is still a challenge for preschoolers because fast food offerings are so high in fat and carbohydrates.

Fast Foods to Avoid

Try to stay away from fast foods. I stayed away from it while I was pregnant. Then the first time I went back, after she was born, I almost threw up from all the grease.

Lauren, 20 – Makayla, 15 months

These foods are absolutely *not* recommended:

- Any meals with more than 30 percent fat content.
- All fried or "crispy" meats or burritos.
- "Double" or "triple" sandwiches.
- Salads with crispy meats or regular salad dressings.
- Most breakfast choices that include meat or eggs are about 50 percent fat.

Be sure to check the nutrition sheets from restaurants offering "Low Carb" or "Low Fat" items. Low Carb dishes are often very high in fat and calories. Low Fat items are often higher in carbohydrates than their regular sisters, and thus may be high in calories.

Tips for Eating Fast foods

I used to eat mostly junk foods. Then I changed and started eating fruits and vegetables instead of the junk from McDonald's® and other fast food places. I was eating more home-cooked meals.

Before, I was eating fast food pretty much every day, once, twice, sometimes three times a day. I was a fast food junkie.

When you try to stop one thing, it's a transaction – so instead of eating fast food I would take a fast food meal away and replace it with something good. Now I probably eat fast food once a month. It was hard and I don't know how I did it. My mom, my brother and sister, we all love fast food.

Anything I ate Emma wanted. So I had to think, do I want her to weigh 300 pounds when she's in high school or do I want her to be healthy?

I was trying to take back roads so I wouldn't see the fast food places on every corner. If it's out of sight, it's out of mind.

I think the only fast food I ate was Arby's® because they were the healthiest fast food place, and it kept me away from the others like McDonald's®.

My family tries not to eat the fast foods. They have seen how I try to keep it away from Emma and they try to do that.

How do you judge fast foods? It depends on the place you go. Some places, if you buy in small portions, it's fine occasionally. But if you're eating fast food four or five times a week, that's going overboard.

> *It's a waste of money. You could save that money . . . within a year I'm sure I spent at least $1000 on fast food (before I got pregnant), and I could have used that money to go on a trip somewhere. Big Mac® – there's at least 900 calories in one burger. The "Super Size Me" movie helped me change.*
>
> *You have to think of yourself and your baby. If you aren't healthy, if you're always lying on the couch eating fast food, then they'll think that's what they should do.*

Paige, 17 – Emma, 10 months

Here are some more tips to add to Paige's suggestions:

- Plan what you will order before you go.
- Pick up the food before you pick up the children.
- If possible, go through a drive-thru window to avoid the tempting sights and smells inside, especially if you are really hungry.
- Take the food home, to a friend's, or a park to avoid temptations.
- Unless you want to be super-sized, avoid that option.
- Occasionally, try a treat such as a milkshake or small fries and divide it among family members. Talk about how it's for a special treat. Perhaps it's someone's birthday, a visit from someone special, or the first day of vacation.

If you decide to cut back on fast food, you'll be doing both yourself and your child a favor. It's a big challenge — *with a huge payoff in better health for both of you.*

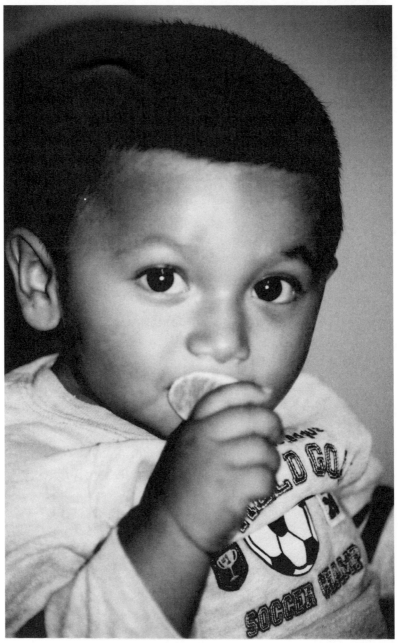

Much of the time he prefers to feed himself.

5

Food Plans
for Picky Toddlers

- **Spoon, Fingers . . .
  or Both**

- **Best to Eat
  Without Wandering**

- **Trying New Foods**

- **Foods She Needs**

- **Providing Choices**

- **Is She a Picky Eater?**

- **Growing a Taste
  for Vegetables**

- **Home-Cooked Is Best**

*Ambika eats carrots and po-
tatoes. She likes banana and
watermelon but not apples.
She eats meat, but she likes
ground beef more than regular
meat. And she likes chicken.*

*I try not to cook with oil.
I add water instead because
the oil is too greasy for her. I
don't add salt or any spices.
She doesn't eat refried beans
or corn, but she likes broccoli
and peas. I cook the broccoli
very soft for her, and sometimes I squish it. I give her
choices so she doesn't feel
pressured.*

Gabrielle, 18 – Ambika, 15 months

*Sometimes he'll go through a stage where he eats
a whole bunch. Other days I have a hard time getting
him to sit down and eat.*

Melinda Jane, 16 – Moises, 15 months

*Agustin is the most pickiest eater. He won't eat any
meat at all. He has low iron, and I have to give him
an iron supplement.*

Trinity, 17 - Agustin, 2

Spoon, Fingers . . . or Both

When your toddler is about a year old, he'll be able to
drink his milk or juice from a small glass or a cup. He's just
beginning to eat with a spoon. By the time a child is a year
old he has learned to eat some foods with his fingers such
as small pieces of bread or cheese. If he has food in his dish
that he really likes, he may still try to eat it with his fingers.

With a little help he'll be more willing to try a spoon. If
you put your hand over his on the spoon, you can help guide
his hand toward his mouth. Do this several times. When he
loses patience, just feed him yourself. At this point you still
need to feed him most of his meal, but soon he'll be able to
do much more himself.

*Makayla eats just about anything that's not too
hard to chew. She loves pasta. I'm trying to gear her
toward eating healthy food like salad and carrots. I
grate the raw carrots. She likes to feed herself. I cut
things up into the size of a penny or smaller so she
can pick it up and hold it. She likes scrambled eggs.*

Lauren, 20 – Makayla, 15 months

Serve your toddler the foods you're eating. You'll need
to make a few changes. He still needs foods that are soft and
chopped or mashed with a fork and foods low in fat. Serve
him foods that are easy to eat and don't require very much
chewing. As he gets older and can chew his food better,

coarsely chopping it will be fine. Soon he will be able to handle bite-size pieces.

Choking hazards for babies and toddlers include:

- **Popcorn**   • **Peas**
- **Hard pieces of raw vegetables and fruits**

Be careful with:

- **Hot dog slices** — Cut thin slices into quarters. (High fat content so don't offer hot dogs often.)
- **Grapes** — Cut in half and they will be fine.
- **Nuts** — Pine nuts and shelled poppy seeds are okay. (See note on page 178 for pine nut/sour cream dip.).

Continue to cut up his meat for a year or so. Cut up other food when possible in chunks he can pick up and eat with his fingers. If you're having garlic bread, he might prefer toast strips. If you're having broccoli, steam it, then cut tiny "trees" for him.

> *Don't let your children control you over what they eat. It's obviously the parent who has the basic choices. If he eats only Easy Mac®, it's the parents' fault. If he doesn't like something, introduce something else – perhaps with bright colors or a different texture.*
>
> Monique, 18 – Ashley, 5 months

You don't need to become a short-order cook. Offer variations of your meals, and include some of his favorites. He might even help you decide what to serve, within your guidelines for nutritious items. If he helps you prepare the food, he's likely to be more willing to eat it.

He may be more interested in eating if your family sits down to eat with him.

Best to Eat without Wandering

One of the most exciting things that happens to a child at about a year is learning how to walk. She likes to practice it

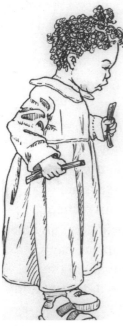

whenever she can. Sooner or later she'll probably try to become a toddling eater. This is not a good idea.

While she may eat some of the food while she moves about, she will most likely set it down here and there. She'll make messes and stain your furniture. Worse, she may finally eat it when it's not very clean, or even slightly spoiled.

There's still another danger. If she stumbled or fell while walking and eating, she could choke on the food. She'll be safer if she learns she must sit and eat only in the place where she is served.

When she's finished eating, there's no need to insist she stay at the table with you. Let her understand that if she gets down, however, she's finished — no coming back to the table again and again for more bites.

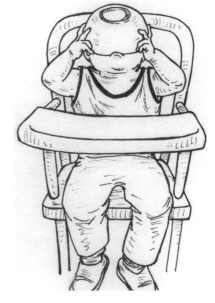

Sometimes parents feed their child in front of the television. Perhaps they think they can get more food into her mouth while she's in a video stupor. This is not a good idea because it teaches her not even to notice what she's eating. She won't learn to enjoy her food, and "unconscious" eating can lead to obesity problems later in her life.

Trying New Foods

Felicia's appetite goes in spurts. She eats a little bit here and there.

Last year when she was one, she wouldn't eat much. I'd make her a plate, usual size for a toddler, and she'd eat maybe half of it.

This year she eats non-stop, then will come back for more.

For snacks she has lots of string cheese and crackers, banana, grapes (I used to cut them in half because of the choking hazard, but now I don't need to). She loves celery and never chokes on it. She also eats it with peanut butter. She started eating peanut butter before she was a year old.

Kristi Ann, 18 – Felicia, 2 1/2

Toddlers should be given only one new food at a time. While some toddlers seem to be able to accept a different food with a new taste or texture quite easily, many don't. Some object to each new flavor or texture that comes along. There are some things you can try that may help.

Don't give him new foods very often. When you do, start with very small portions and serve it with other foods that he likes to eat.

It may help if he eats with the family. If he sees that others are eating this new food and even seem to enjoy it, he may be more likely to try it. If he still won't eat it, tell him to eat just a spoonful so he'll know what it's like. He may have to try this food many times before he decides to eat it.

Keep food portions small. Large servings may discourage him. Toddlers have small appetites and small stomachs. They only want a small portion because that is all they can eat.

The appropriate portion for toddlers is 1/4 slice of bread,

and 2 tablespoons of rice, potatoes or pasta. He needs only 1/4 cup of fruit and 1/4 cup of vegetables. All serving sizes will seem small. He can have more if he wants it.

Foods She Needs

On pp. 99-100 is the MyPyramid for Kids. This is designed for children aged 2 and older. Your toddler needs about the same foods, only smaller portions. We'll talk more about MyPyramid for Kids in the next chapter.

Foods rich in protein are important for healthy growth and development. Proteins are found in dairy products (milk, yogurt, and cheese), poultry, soy, dry beans, and eggs. She also needs lean red meats and iron-fortified cereals to get the necessary iron. Fruits and vegetables rich in vitamin C such as citrus fruits, strawberries, broccoli, cantaloupe, and fruit juices are important to help with the absorption of iron.

Some children have a hard time eating meat, especially the red meats. Sometimes serving chopped fruits or applesauce with the meats will help her eat them. For example, a little applesauce on the spoon with the meat could make the meat seem less dry and easier to chew or swallow.

Fish is a good source of protein but some small children are allergic to shellfish. If you want to serve shellfish to your child, check with your healthcare provider.

She also needs a variety of green and yellow vegetables to get all the necessary vitamins. Some children develop strong feelings against eating vegetables later on. The vegetables she gets used to eating now may help her avoid this problem.

If it's something he hasn't tried, Enriko will say, "No." Then I try it, and I say, "This is good, mmm . . . this is delicious." Then he puts it in his mouth

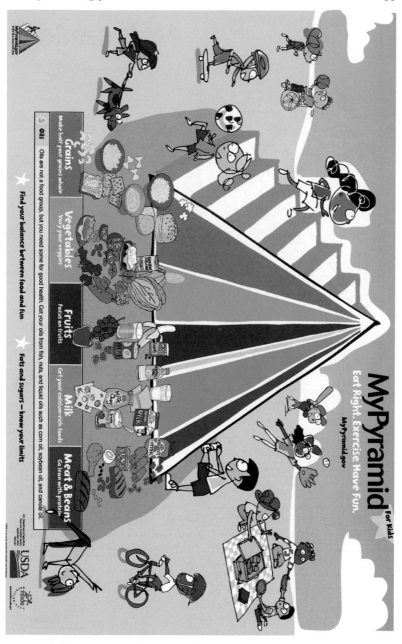

MyPyramid for Kids provides specifics on healthy eating.

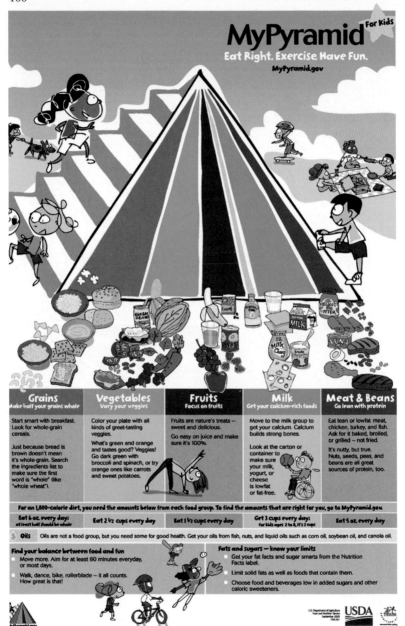

*Any time you want a reminder of the various foods your child needs,
each day, check out MyPyramid for Kids.*

and mimics me, and starts eating it.
    *Enriko usually eats at the same time everyone else
does, at the table.*

                                    Delores, 18 – Enriko, 2½

Toddlers need to have whole milk. She needs the calories
from whole milk, so this is not a good time for skim or low
fat milk. Other calcium-rich foods are yogurt, cheese, and
calcium-fortified foods and juices.

At this age children also need some fats. It is important
to get the essential oils. A tablespoon of oil in food preparation works well (either soy, canola, safflower, or olive oil).
A salad dressing dip can be used instead.

Vitamin E that is needed for healthy growth is found in
many of the foods that also provide the essential fatty acids.
Salmon, light chunk tuna, and spinach are examples.

Your child is more likely to eat and to develop good
eating habits if the television is off and loud music is not
playing. It helps her pay more attention to eating.

*Sometimes my grandparents go in the front room
while Felicia and I sit at the table, but usually we try
to eat together.*
    *I notice Felicia eats more when we're all there.
She's more focused and knows where we are. We talk,
they ask about my day, and they ask Felicia about her
day at school.*

                                                Kristi Ann

Providing Choices

*I don't think you should make a child eat when he
doesn't want to. Sometimes Alyssa doesn't want to eat.
To force somebody to eat isn't good.*
    *You need to give them different things to taste. If
you give them the same thing every day or just fast
food, that's not good.*

*Alyssa won't eat a new food until she sees me
eating it. But when she tries it, she usually likes it.*

Chloe, 22 – Alyssa, 2; Denae, 1

A toddler often has strong feelings about food. He wants
to decide what he is going to eat as well as how much he
eats. Let him make some of these decisions. As long as he is
only offered healthy foods, he will most likely make good
choices. He will probably end up with a fairly good diet
if heavy desserts, candy or soft drinks are not among the
choices available. His menu may not be the one you would
have chosen, but it may be adequate.

If you worry about his eating, keep a record for a week.
Write down everything he consumes. Then analyze his
intake. By the time he's two, each day he needs:

- **2 cups milk**
- **1 cup each, fruits and vegetables**
- **3 ounces bread and cereal**
- **2 ounces protein foods**
- **small amount of "good" fat or oil (No *trans* fat!)**

Remember, serving sizes for toddlers are small. Analyze
the food he's eaten through your written record. Perhaps he
ate a generous amount of meat one night, then refused the
protein you served the next night. Did he eat several fruits
and vegetables that day? Over the week, did he eat foods
from each food group? If so, he's probably coming
along nicely.

If you feel his dietary needs are simply not being met,
talk to the doctor or nutritionist at WIC about vitamin pills.

Is She a Picky Eater?

*Madison used to be a picky eater. I tried to feed her
good healthy stuff, but she wouldn't eat. For awhile,*

my stepmother would coax her to eat something. Now
when she gives me a hard time, I just walk away and
see what she eats. I don't want to be saying over and
over, "Madison, eat, eat."

If she's not hungry, I'm not going to force her.
                                    Kaitlyn, 16 – Madison, 2

Toddlers have a reputation for being picky eaters. There
may be several reasons:

She eats junk food. Her stomach is too small to add the
nutritious foods she needs on top of the junk. If she's eating
candy, cookies, or other junk food, she won't have the
appetite for the foods she needs.

If she's a picky eater, don't offer sweets at all. For her
snacks, offer such foods as carrots, graham crackers, apples,
milk, or peaches.

She should not have raw carrot sticks until she's past
three because of the danger of choking. She could eat carrot
sticks that have been cooked until they are slightly soft. If
you grate raw carrots for her, she can pick up a handful and
eat them
herself with-
out risk.

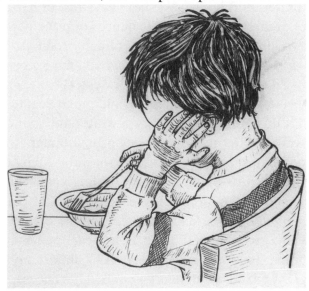

Remem-
ber that raw
vegetables
have at
least as
much, usu-
ally more,
nutrition
than cooked
ones. If she
likes to eat
frozen peas

but not cooked ones, that's okay.

She's becoming very independent. For a parent to try to be in charge of a toddler's eating is almost always a losing battle. Put nutritious food in front of her, in small servings. Be sure she sees you eating these foods with pleasure. If she doesn't want something, suggest a tiny bite, but don't bribe or try to force her. If she doesn't like it, don't worry. Encourage her to taste that food again next time you serve it. She may decide it tastes good after a number of tries.

> *Salvador likes apples and peanut butter — he dips the apple into the peanut butter. He started eating peanut butter at my mom's house. She loves peanut butter and jelly sandwiches. When the peanut butter got stuck in the top of his mouth, she suggested apple slices.*
>
> Katrina, 18 – 7 months pregnant; Salvador, 19 months

Does she like peanut butter? If you spread peanut butter thinly on one slice of bread and serve it with a glass of milk for her morning snack, she'll have one of her three portions of grains, one of her three ounces of protein, and one of her two cups (or the equivalent) of dairy food. Add some grated carrots and a piece of fruit, and you have a healthy lunch — she may forget she's a picky eater!

Note: A few children are allergic to peanuts. If your child has this problem, or it runs in your family, of course you'll be very careful about serving peanut butter to her.

Yogurt is a tasty substitute for milk. Many children prefer fruit yogurts to plain yogurt. Adding your own fruit to plain yogurt may not only taste better, but it's also a good way to avoid the added sugar in many commercial fruit yogurts. Fresh strawberries, blueberries, peaches, bananas, mango, grapes (cut in half), applesauce — almost any fruit tastes great mixed with yogurt — or cottage cheese.

Note: If you use canned fruit, throw out the syrup that comes with the fruit before you use it. When you're buying canned fruit, choose the unsweetened variety. Fruit by itself is already sweet.

The trick is to think about the foods she likes, then create combinations that she'll want to eat. It's okay if she eats nothing but cheese and whole-grain crackers, peaches, peas, and maybe a little canned tuna or chicken for days.

You know how toddlers like routine. For example, she probably has a set bedtime routine. She may not want frequent changes in her food either.

A picky toddler could be insulted if he's offered an entire meal of "strange" things. Always include foods he likes. Simply place a small amount of the new food on his plate without making a big deal about it. And remember how small toddler portions are compared to what you consider a serving for you.

Growing a Taste for Vegetables

Many children like vegetables, but others don't. It's the same for adults. If you don't eat vegetables much, and don't really like them, know that it's not a genetic trait that is necessarily passed on to your child. This distaste for vegetables can be changed!

I'm a picky eater and I'm surprised Kendall isn't. I don't eat vegetables at all. When she eats broccoli, I won't eat it.

My family told me to have an open mind. They said, "Just because you don't like vegetables doesn't mean Kendall won't. Make it and she can try it."

Like the steamed broccoli. I don't eat it but I make it for her. I learned this when my little cousin at a Chinese restaurant was eating broccoli and Kendall wanted to try it.

She said, "What's that?" and she grabbed it. She tried it and she liked it. She was about 21/2 then.

Ukari, 18 - Kendall, 3

Kendall decided to eat broccoli in spite of her mom's negative expectations. Your child is more likely to eat vegetables, however, if you eat them with him. If you, like Ukari, don't much like vegetables, you might tell your child you're going to experiment with him.

Then go ahead and serve various kinds of vegetables, and both of you follow that at-least-one-taste philosophy for ten times. You and your child may end up getting those valuable nutrients so prevalent in vegetables.

First of all, don't start out assuming he won't eat broccoli or green beans or peas or . . . Begin by steaming the vegetable. As mentioned in chapter 3, put the vegetables in the steamer basket, add about 1/2" of water to the pan, and cover. Your vegetables will cook as they steam.

Steamed vegetables retain more nutrients than they would simply being boiled. The valuable vitamins and minerals are less likely to wash away in the cooking water. Most of us think steamed vegetables taste better, too.

Try different cooking times. Perhaps your child prefers well-cooked, soft broccoli. Or he likes still-crisp and bright green broccoli better. So often the style in which you serve foods makes a difference. Mashed cauliflower looks a lot like mashed potatoes. Baked sweet potato may appeal more to him than squash.

Occasionally do special things to make meals fun. Make a face on a plate with cherry tomatoes, green pepper, and carrots. Cook pancakes in weird shapes, perhaps his initials. He might like dipping pretzels and fruit slices into yogurt. Even setting your table with bright placemats and inexpensive dishes with a child motif may intrigue him.

Home-Cooked Is Best

Zoltan eats what I eat. For breakfast sometimes I fix eggs and toast. I bought him toddler cereal and he eats that a lot. He likes grits and cream of wheat. He likes yogurt, fruit flavored, and he loves pancakes.

He likes vegetables – peas, broccoli, cauliflower, Brussels sprouts. I don't give him corn yet.

Catava, 19 – Zoltan, 17 months; Bikita, 5 months

Cooking the food yourself generally results in more nutritious dishes than you get using convenience foods. Canned soup, for example, is extremely high in salt, and your toddler doesn't need a lot of salt. Processed foods also contain a variety of preservatives, colorings, and artificial flavorings. Serving them once in a while is all right. Having an already-prepared food frequently is not especially good for any of us. Neither, of course, are fast foods.

Even if the food is made especially for toddlers, it may not be very nutritious. *Check the label!*

Did you realize that hot dogs are not very good for toddlers? Even if the skin is split or they are cut into little slices, he could choke on them. As for food value, hot dogs are very high in fat.

If your toddler doesn't want to eat a food he needs, what else might have the same nutritive value? If he doesn't drink much milk, put milk in puddings and soups. If he likes cheese, it will provide many of the same nutrients as milk. So will cottage cheese and yogurt. Cheese can also take the place of meat some of the time.

By the time he's two, your child will need much the same food as older preschoolers. See the next chapter for more suggestions.

Learning to eat a wide variety of nutritious foods when he's a toddler will benefit your child throughout his life.

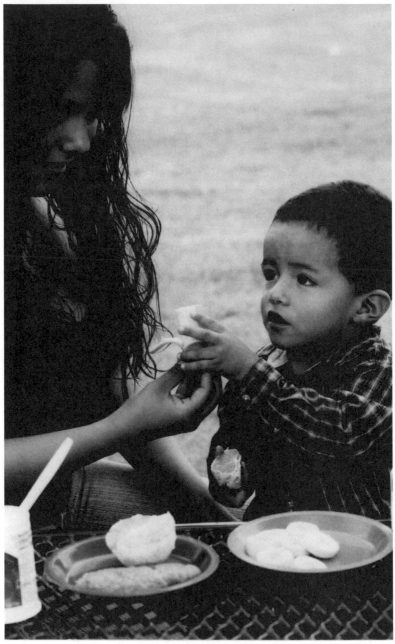

He likes to eat with Mom (or Dad).

6

She's a Preschooler — You're Her Model

I don't like shrimp but Kendall does. I cook it because she and my husband like it. I just pretend I'm eating it because if Kendall sees me not eating it, she will think it's nasty.

Feeding her what I don't like is hard. I try to eat in front of her but I just don't like some things. If she's eating something I don't like, I serve myself something else. If they're eating rice and shrimp, I eat rice and beans.

Kendall also likes tuna and I don't. She likes tuna with crackers and on tostadas.

Ukari, 19 – Kendall, 3

He Likes Eating with His Family

By this age, eating together works well because by now your preschooler probably eats many of the same foods as the rest of the family. Now he needs a lot less help than he did earlier. He's skillful at handling his fork, spoon, and glass.

Sometimes he still needs help, with cutting his meat in small pieces, for example. But now he eats independently, and he seldom spills his milk or makes a huge mess — unlike the typical two-year-old.

Your preschooler will enjoy eating with you and the rest of your family. Sitting down together to eat, with loud music and the TV turned off, is a great way to talk together. When he hears Mom, Dad, and other family members discuss the day's happenings, he'll feel a part of his family unit. He, too, may like sharing his day.

> *We all eat together — my mom, dad, my two broth-ers and me and the kids. It feels better to all sit down and eat at the same time.*
>
> Dakarai, 20 - Gazali, 3; Julisha, 1 1/2

When you ask your child a question — and wait for his answer — he will feel he's truly part of the group. He may even be willing to stay at the table longer because he's enjoying being with you.

We don't advocate insisting that a child under 5 stay at the table until others finish eating. Sitting there is hard for an active child.

Assure him that when he's finished he can go play. With this policy, he's more likely to be cooperative while he's sitting at the table.

When he eats with his family, a preschooler, just like a toddler, will notice that others eat the various foods served. Of course most children are not going to mimic *all* these good eating habits. They're more likely to try a food, however, if Mommy or Daddy likes it.

> *I like seafood and pasta. I don't like sweet peas, broccoli, or cauliflower, but Zaila does. She comes home from school and says, "Mommy, I want sweet peas."*
>
> *I hate scrambled eggs, but she loves them, so I fix them for her.*
>
> Jasmine, 19 - Zaila, 3; Cody, 7 months

Many families have a policy of asking everyone (this rule needs to apply to parents too!) to take a bite of each food. Perhaps it's only one pea. Extending the policy to include trying each food ten times may mean your picky eater learns to enjoy a wider variety of foods.

Are You a Good Example?

In some families, asking the child to eat everything the parents eat is not good. Do you eat French fries and other high fat foods? Do you have a "sweet tooth" and enjoy cookies, candy, sugared cereal, and other foods containing lots of sugar?

Foods high in fat and sugar will cause her, like the rest of us, to gain extra weight. If your child eats these foods, she's going to feel full too soon. She'll be less likely to eat the fruits, vegetables, and whole grains she needs.

Another problem with the sweet foods is their effect on her teeth. That "sweet tooth" too often turns into teeth filled with painful cavities. These cavities will be costly to fix. In some families, the cavities aren't treated, simply because there is no money and no insurance for dental care.

> *She says her teeth hurt. She has never been to a dentist, but she says it hurts. She likes soda, probably has it once a day.*

*She likes to eat candy. Sometimes her grand-
parents give her more candy. I try to talk to them but
they don't listen.*

Emmy, 21 – Zalena, 3 1/2

Emmy really needs to get Zalena to a dentist. Experienc-
ing pain in her teeth undoubtedly means Zalena has dental
cavities. They need to be fixed immediately, whether they
are baby or permanent teeth.

Soda is very bad for teeth, and candy certainly doesn't
help Zalena. Do you ever have this problem? You don't
want your child to eat candy or other unhealthy foods, but
Grandma insists, "Just a little won't hurt her."

Remember that your child's grandparents love your child
dearly. They want her to be healthy now and in the future.
Perhaps you and Dad can tactfully help them understand
how important it is that your child eat healthy foods. They
can show their love in lots of ways without resorting to
giving her candy.

In fact, your discussion might go better if you offer to
forego most of the sweet foods yourself.

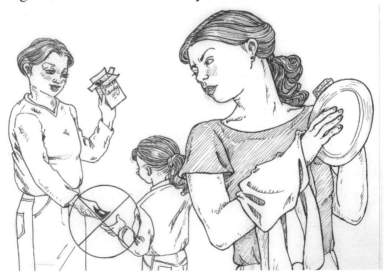

So What's Healthy for a Preschooler?

See pp. 99-100 for the U.S. Department of Agriculture's MyPyramid for Kids. MyPyramid contains a rainbow of colored vertical stripes which represent the five food groups plus fats and oils. Use this website, **<mypyramid.gov/kids>** for more excellent nutrition information. This site even has a game, coloring sheet, and poster you can download.

Notice the stairsteps with a little girl walking up, signifying the need for exercise every day. MyPyramid is an excellent guide to planning the foods you'll offer your preschooler and to remind you of the importance of exercise.

What counts as one portion? Recommended portions for young children are quite small. No McDonald's® Quarter-Pounders® here!

You may find it's not difficult to provide all these basic foods when you count three meals and at least two snacks each day. You'll want to find which foods in each food group appeal to your youngster.

This means if he doesn't appear to like something you'd like him to eat, you experiment with different ways of fixing that food. You also look for other foods in that food group that he does like.

Dairy Foods — More than Milk

As a starter, your preschooler needs two portions a day of dairy foods. Does she like milk? Simply drinking two cups of milk meets this requirement. Or replace a cup of milk with 1 1/2 ounces of natural cheese (such as Cheddar) or two ounces of processed cheese (such as American). Does she like string cheese? Great! There's another dairy food.

Does she like chocolate milk better than plain? This is fine, assuming she's not getting too many calories from eating candy and cookies. And thinking of calories — by the time she's 3, it's okay to offer 2 or 1 percent milk. She

needed whole milk when she switched from breast milk or
formula to glasses of milk.

If you move gradually from whole milk to 2 percent, then
to 1 percent, she, and you, may find the "new" kind of milk
tastes just as good. Most important, you're cutting back on
the fat in your child's diet as well as your own.

Protein Builds Bodies

Zalena likes vegetables and fruit. She eats carrots,
broccoli. The only thing she doesn't like is meat. She
doesn't eat any at all.

She eats cheese. She drinks milk in the morning,
and again at night with cookies.

Emmy

Some children don't like to eat meat. Don't worry. Keep
offering it, but remember that the meat/protein group also
includes eggs, peanut butter, tofu, dried beans and legumes.
Four-year-olds need three or four ounces a day of foods rich
in protein.

If your child likes meat, a portion means only two or
three ounces of lean meat, poultry or fish, a portion about
the size of a deck of cards.

Your preschooler probably prefers meats that are easy to
chew. Tender meat thinly sliced across the grain is likely to
appeal to him. He still may like for you to cut his chicken
into small pieces. Mixing meat into sauces for macaroni or
noodles is a good choice. Or mix the meat into soup.

If he doesn't like meat, serve other foods high in protein.
But continue offering very small servings of the various
meats you eat. Some day he may decide meat is worth
eating after all.

Making soup with dried beans adds protein. If he doesn't
like the texture of beans, puree the beans in the blender after
they're thoroughly cooked. Then add other soup ingredients.

If he eats a cup of lentil soup, he'll have the equivalent of two ounces of meat. A soy or bean burger patty provides about an ounce. So does 1/4 cup cooked dried beans, an egg, a tablespoon of peanut butter, or a small handful of nuts or seeds.

Note: If he doesn't like meat, realize that there's overlap between the milk and meat group. Milk, cheese and yogurt are all rich in protein.

If he doesn't eat red meat, he might not be getting enough iron in his food although eggs, chicken, whole grains, and dark green vegetables also contain iron. Does he take vitamins? Check the bottle for iron content. His vitamins probably contain at least some of the iron he needs.

Making Vegetables Appetizing

I think kids want to eat vegetables, I really do. I think they aren't always given the opportunity to eat them. They don't have to be cooked.

Almost every day I have a cold plate in the refrigerator with raw vegetables, and I bring it out every day about 11 a.m., and it sets out for several hours with ranch dressing. And everyone that passes by takes something.

I don't think parents try vegetables enough.

Hannah, 23 – Mackenzie, 41/2

While many children like vegetables and eat them readily, the vegetable group is probably the one most often rejected. Trying to get her to eat even three small portions, a total of 1 1/2 cups daily, may be a challenge.

Many children don't like the textures in some vegetables. Try serving them in different ways. A child who objects to the texture of cooked carrots may accept thin carrot sticks. Bean sprouts, both raw and cooked, are often fun vegetables for young children.

Spreading peanut butter on celery pieces gives her both a protein and a vegetable. If she spreads the peanut butter on the celery herself, she may like it even better. (Toddlers need their celery steamed for a couple of minutes to avoid the risk of choking.)

Often it's not easy to find a way she'll like, but it's worth the effort. Children need to learn to eat veggies. Those vitamins and minerals are extremely important to their health.

> **Note:** Insisting she eat her whole serving of broccoli if she says she doesn't like it is likely to backfire. She'll resist even more next time.

Around 4 or 5 years your child may like a small salad. Offer lettuce with a little salad dressing.

Another time she may want her salad made of unbroken small leaves of lettuce and a little salad dressing she can put on herself.

Or perhaps she'll prefer no salad dressing at all.

Remember — these preferences may change daily.

Raw Veggies Are Fine

Of course you don't have to cook many of the vegetables if he prefers them raw. Most children like thin carrot sticks, and may move on to raw broccoli florets, cauliflower pieces, radishes, zucchini, jicama, and others.

Vanesa feels strongly that eating should be fun — in the context of offering nutritious food.

> *If you cut things out in cartoon shapes . . . like cucumbers. I cut cucumber slices in fish shapes. Then I had Andrea dip them in a non-fat salad dressing I colored blue.*
>
> *I told her the fish were swimming, and she had a great time eating cucumbers.*
>
> Vanesa, 19 - Andrea, 4; Josefina, 8 months

She may like a bowl of frozen peas better than the cooked ones the rest of the family eats. That's okay, too.

When Mackenzie says, "I don't like it," I say, "You never had it."

"Well, I had it at my dad's house."

"That doesn't count. That wasn't here." She is slowly learning that doesn't work. We insist she try it, like one tiny pea.

She loves peas now. If I take them out of the freezer, "Can I have a bowl of them frozen?"

Even my boyfriend said, "She can't eat them frozen!"

I say, "Why not?"

I think a lot of parents expect their kids not to like vegetables. They don't all have to be cooked.

Parents need to pick their battles. Do we need to argue about whether to eat the vegetables cooked or raw?

Hannah

If he's picky about eating vegetables, let him try dipping chunks of vegetables in a little ranch dressing. Give him raw, slightly cooked, or well-cooked vegetables, whichever he prefers. Or offer a small bowl of salad dressing made with canola or olive oil. The essential oils in the salad dressing make it a healthy choice for him.

Sometimes Neena eats vegetables only two or three days in a week.

Tonight I'm fixing steamed vegetables, and she can eat pieces with ranch dressing. She likes that.

Fidelia, 19 – Neena, 3

Adding grated carrots or finely chopped bell peppers to hamburger, spaghetti sauce, taco meat, or dipping sauce is another way to add veggies to your meals.

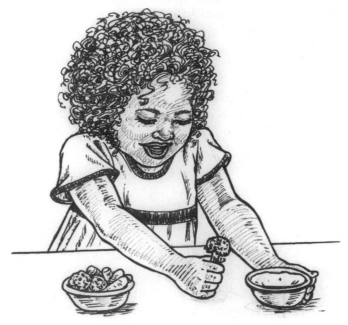

Let him help you prepare vegetables. He probably can't use a knife safely yet, but he can wash those vegetables. He'll need a sturdy step stool. You may want to limit the amount of water in the sink. (This is not the time to flood the kitchen.)

Fruits Are Easy

Kendall will try anything, but she loves fruit. She would rather eat fruit than any other food.

                                                              Ukari

Eating two or three portions of fruit each day is easy for most children (providing it's readily available to them). One portion is an apple, peach, orange, or 1/2 cup berries.

She probably likes fruit juices. Be sure the "juice" you offer her is 100 percent real juice. Fruit juice drinks are not a good substitute. They contain too much sugar and too little juice. Even with 100 percent juices, 3/4 cup of juice each day is enough. The whole fruits are better for her.

When she's thirsty, encourage her to drink water.

There are many wonderful fruits that taste good and are good for her. Bananas, apples cored and thinly sliced, orange sections, melon balls or chunks, peaches, nectarines, mangos, berries, and apricots, for example. You can also serve her well-drained canned fruit. As mentioned before, choose the cans of unsweetened fruit.

> *Neena may have a mango and/or a banana in the morning, or I'll make her a shake with strawberries and banana.*
>
> Fidelia

Giving her a fruit for breakfast, perhaps sliced on her oatmeal or cold cereal, is a good eye-opener. Another fruit at lunch, and she's already eaten the recommended two fruits for the day.

Fruits also make excellent — and delicious — desserts.

Whole Grains for Fiber, B Vitamins

Your child probably enjoys the grain group — breads, cereal, rice, pasta, tortillas, pita, etc. By age 4, he needs four or five portions each day from this group, according to My-Pyramid for Kids. An ounce translates to one piece of bread, 1/2 cup cooked cereal, rice or pasta, or one cup cold cereal.

It's important to choose whole-grain cereals, breads, pasta, and tortillas, and to use brown rice instead of white. They provide fiber, minerals (magnesium, iron, and zinc), and important B vitamins for your child.

> *I like pasta and Mackenzie loves it. I fix pasta salad with vegetables, black olives, and cheese chunks. It's always whole grain pasta. Even our macaroni and cheese, it's the whole grain macaroni. Some stores have an organic section and that's where you can get the whole grain mix for macaroni and cheese.*
>
> Hannah

Your child gets a good start on his day with a breakfast that includes whole-grain food. Given, you probably don't have a lot of time to fix breakfast for yourself and your child. But do you know that "instant" oatmeal cooks in the microwave in less than two minutes?

Try adding raisins or dried cranberries before cooking it. Or slice a banana over the hot cereal and add a little milk. Or slice peaches, strawberries, mango, actually almost any fresh fruit that your child enjoys. He may decide he wants two fruits on his oatmeal. Already he has eaten his two portions of fruit along with the serving of grain.

If you choose whole grain breads, crackers, and tortillas, offering four more whole grain servings to your child's meals and snacks during the day should be no problem. Perhaps a sandwich at lunch (two slices of bread), whole grain crackers for a snack, maybe include brown rice at dinner — and lo and behold, he's eaten his five portions of grain.

Breakfast Is Important

Research shows clearly that children who skip breakfast don't do as well in school. They simply don't have the morning energy they get from a good breakfast. They also are likely to behave better if they eat a good breakfast.

You may have very little time to cook breakfast. But please don't skip this important meal. If your child skips breakfast, is it possible she hasn't been offered something that tastes good to her? It's also important that breakfast items be nutritious and easy to eat.

Try to plan an extra 15 minutes to sit down with your child as both of you eat breakfast. Actually, many children are hungriest in the morning, less hungry at lunch, and may have very little appetite by evening. Going along with this pattern can become a healthy custom.

As someone said, "Ideally, we'd all eat like a king at

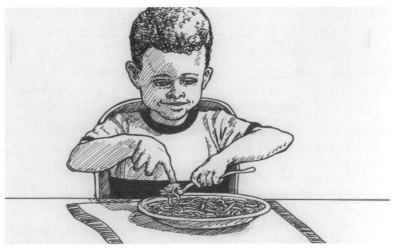

breakfast, a prince at lunch, and a pauper at dinner!"

*One of the main problems I have is for breakfast
there aren't many nutritious things. For cereal there's
all the sugar coated, marshmallow stuff. You'd think
there'd be more breakfast things high in nutrition.*

*Now they're even coming up with Cheerios® with
yogurt and sugar on them. Or they stick something
extra in the oatmeal. We buy the regular oatmeal and
put the fruit in it.*

Vanesa

Don't feel limited by traditional breakfast foods. A nutritious, delicious breakfast can be cereal and fruit or eggs
and whole grain toast. But think beyond these typical early
morning foods. Would she like a cheese sandwich? Put
cheese between two slices of whole grain bread. Heat about
25 seconds in the microwave. She may devour it happily.

Nutritious leftovers she likes can make a great breakfast.
Rice, beans and tortillas for example. Or a small serving
of tuna casserole or whole-grain pasta with sauce. And of
course there's always peanut butter toast. Occasionally she
might even have a piece of leftover pizza for breakfast.

If she likes dry cereal, carefully select the kind you buy. Many dry cereals contain no whole grain, and have far too much sugar in them. You probably offered Cheerios® to your baby when she was about six months old. That's when she was learning to pick up food and stuff it in her mouth.

That was a good choice providing the Cheerios® didn't have added sugar in them. Many of the cereals advertised for children contain far too much sugar. Read the label.

It's good to check labels. Calories are not necessarily bad for children because they're still growing, but little kids don't need the portions we need.

Veda, 18 - Mesha, 3

Notice the difference between the Apple Jacks® and the oatmeal labels below. The oatmeal contains no sugar while the Apple Jacks®, like many cereals advertised to children, has a lot — 16 grams or 17/9 tablespoons of sugar. This translates to 80 calories, 61 percent of the total!

Nutrition Facts

Serving Size 1 Cup (33g/1.2 oz.)
Servings Per Container   About 13

Amount Per Serving	Cereal	Cereal with ½ Cup Vitamins A&D Fat Free Milk
Calories	130	170
Calories from Fat	5	5
	% Daily Value**	
Total Fat 0.5g*	1%	1%
Saturated Fat 0g	0%	0%
Trans Fat 0g		
Cholesterol 0mg	0%	0%
Sodium 150mg	6%	9%
Potassium 35mg	1%	7%
Total Carbohydrate 30g	10%	12%
Dietary Fiber 1g	4%	4%
Sugars 16g		
Other Carbohydrate 13g		
Protein 1g		

Apple Jacks® label

Nutrition Facts

Serving Size ½ cup (40g dry)
Servings Per Container about 13

Amount Per Serving	Cereal
Calories	150
Calories from Fat	25
	% Daily Value*
Total Fat 2.5g	4%
Saturated Fat 0.5g	3%
Polyunsaturated Fat 1g	
Monounsaturated Fat 1g	
Cholesterol 0mg	0%
Sodium 0mg	0%
Total Carbohydrate 27g	9%
Dietary Fiber 4g	16%
Soluble Fiber 1g	
Insoluble Fiber 2g	
Sugars 0g	
Protein 5g	

Oatmeal label

If more than 25 percent of the calories in a cereal are from sugar, that food needs to be considered dessert, not a whole grain.

Many brands of cereal that lots of children eat are more than half sugar. Your preschooler does not need it. If you prefer to serve her cold cereal, find those made of whole grains and containing very little sugar. You may need to try several to find one she likes.

Cooked oatmeal and hot wheat cereal are usually healthier for a child — and more economical.

Simple Menu Ideas

Whole grain hot or cold cereal with fruit makes a great breakfast. For his mid-morning snack, offer him a piece of toast lightly spread with his favorite jam or peanut butter along with a glass of milk.

At lunch he might have a sandwich. If his sandwich contains cheese, or perhaps chicken, and he adds carrot sticks and a glass of milk to his meal, he's well on his way to getting the day's nutrients.

Is he hungry at mid-afternoon? Offer whole-wheat crackers and apple slices. For dinner, you might serve brown rice, a small serving of fish, a vegetable such as green beans, and perhaps a small salad.

There you have it. He's had his two cups of milk (or equivalent), three portions each of fruit and vegetables, plenty of protein, and five portions of whole grain foods.

There are lots of ways to offer the basic foods to your child. These suggestions are provided only to give you a start in figuring out what your child likes to eat from each essential food group. Then it's your challenge to create a daily food plan for him that includes all these groups.

More power to you! *You're giving your preschooler a great start.*

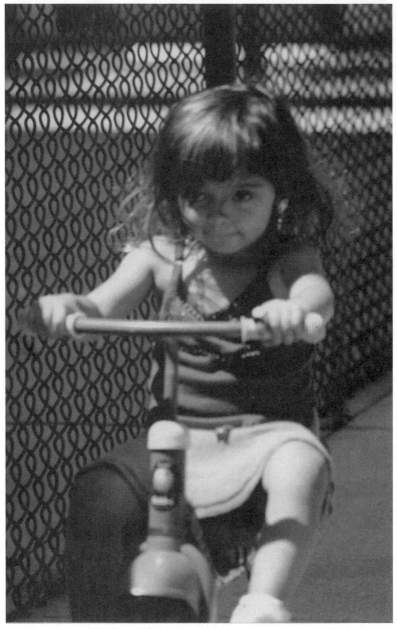

She's getting plenty of exercise
so she's not likely to gain too much weight.

7

Fat-Proofing Your Child

Yes, I worry about Ambika getting fat. Later on I'm afraid she'll experience all those fast foods and all those greasy foods out there, and she's going to want them.

I'll cook for her here, and make her know there's always food here. She won't have to go to fast foods. I'll give her options as to what she wants me to cook.

Gabrielle, 18 – Ambika, 15 months

I learned a lot in my parenting classes, like eating healthy. I think that's neat, even learning how the advertising on TV gets the kids to want stuff like Fruit Loops®, makes them all look good. But it's nothing but a whole bunch of sugar.

Ameera, 17 – Aida, 12 months

Effects of Poor Choices

The world of food and nutrition is filled with information about what we should and shouldn't eat. Advertisements on TV, radio, and billboards tell us to eat this or that because it is good for us or because we like it. We also have new information about the results of poor eating choices.

In the United States more and more children and adults are overweight. Even many young children are extremely overweight. Is this a health problem? Or is being fat simply a matter of appearance?

Indeed yes, being overweight can be a problem whether you're 3, 17, or 60. And appearance is not the major difficulty. A fat child can't run fast or play as actively as a thinner person. He may get teased because of his weight. He may have other emotional and physical problems. He is more likely to develop asthma, for example.

A child who is overweight is more likely to become an obese adult with significantly higher risk of heart disease, diabetes, and other diseases.

Weight matters a lot. If your child becomes very overweight, his health will be affected.

My friend who is 18 has a two-year-old son. He drinks soda all the time and eats fried stuff. He's chunky, not healthy-chunky, just fat-chunky.

My mom had diabetes. How I feed Luis now is going to affect his future. There are a bunch of illnesses out there that people get because of how they eat.

Carlota, 18 – Luis, 41/2

You can do a lot to keep your child from developing these problems. Perhaps the most important thing is to be a good model. If you eat mainly foods high in nutrients and low in sugar and fat, your child is likely to follow your example. If you seldom eat French fries, you won't be tempted to give them to your toddler.

Overweight children usually don't eat a healthy diet, and they are not as active as they should be for good health. Many children spend several hours in front of the television or computer each day. Not only are they not playing actively, they may be eating snacks high in sugar and fat. On the TV they see hundreds of flashy food ads, many for fast foods, sodas, and other poor food choices. And Dad or Mom may sometimes be a poor example:

> *His dad eats a lot of candy. Whatever his dad eats, Salvador eats.*
>
> *Whenever we go to the store, I give Salvador candy and he loves it. He eats a lot of potato chips and cereal without the milk.*
> Katrina, 18 – 7 months pregnant; Salvador, 19 months

Danger of Diabetes

One of the key concerns for overweight children and adults is the development of diabetes, a disease that affects the body's utilization of sugar. There are three common types of diabetes.

- **Insulin-dependent (type I)** Once called juvenile diabetes because it began in childhood, this type relies on insulin being injected every day.

- **Noninsulin-dependent (type II)** used to be called maturity-onset diabetes because it affected older adults. It can be controlled by a careful diet and exercise program. Sometimes insulin is required.

- **Gestational diabetes** occurs during pregnancy and usually disappears after the birth of the baby. About 50 percent of women who experience this condition may develop type II diabetes within five to ten years. It can be controlled by diet and exercise.

I had gestational diabetes and I had to watch my diet very strictly. I had to go to a dietician and she coached me on everything. She told me how to figure out the nutrition on the label.

My mom thought it was a little ridiculous and not that important, but I knew how bad this could be. She didn't really think I had diabetes because I didn't need insulin, probably because I kept on the diet.

Danté was 6 pounds 7 ounces, so I had a natural birth, pretty easy actually, only 81/2 hours of labor.

Argentina, 18 – Danté, 6 months

Researchers say that the tendency for diabetes is present at birth. Type I is believed to be caused by a complex autoimmune process. In people who are at risk for type II diabetes, being overweight can be the cause because excess fat keeps insulin produced in the body from working properly.

In the last few years concern has grown among both professionals and families because there is a great increase in type II diabetes among school-age children. At the same time there is a great increase in obesity among young children. A diet high in fat and sugar combined with a lack of exercise is the cause.

These are the perfect conditions for developing diabetes. Maybe you or your child won't get diabetes now, but the habits of poor eating and lack of exercise are hard to change. If that lifestyle goes on for a long time, the risk increases. You don't want that to happen.

Madison loves candy and sweets, but my step-
mother and I agreed that she shouldn't have too much.
We don't want her to get diabetes. Once a day she has
a Popsicle.

Kaitlyn, 16 – Madison, 2

Steps to a Healthier Body

There are two equally important steps to becoming your healthiest self and to helping your child grow up as a naturally healthy person — exercise and diet. (Of course "diet" refers to what we eat, and doesn't simply mean to diet to lose weight.)

Let's consider exercise first. While you're pregnant, you may find it hard to exercise. Some easy ways to get yourself moving are:

- Wait on yourself. Don't ask someone else to get something for you. Get up and get it.

- Leave the TV remote by the TV. Want to change the channel? Ah, more exercise.

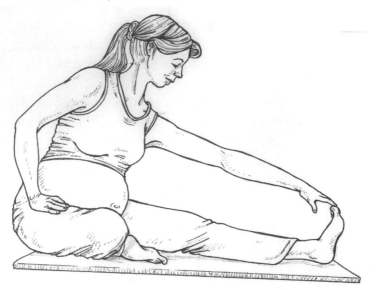

- Park the car at least 5 minutes walk from the store or school. Or ask the person driving to let you off a block or two from your destination.
- Take a walk during your break or lunchtime.
- Maybe your neighborhood isn't always safe for walk-ing. Think about places you can walk for ten minutes or so. Maybe it's a mall, a library, at school, or a friend or relative's neighborhood that will work for you.

Exercise makes you feel better. You feel better when you go out for a walk — and it gives you something to brag about.

I swam as much as I could. It feels real good to sit there in the water. And it's so relaxing when you move your joints and it's effortless. Usually you're real hot when you're pregnant, and the water feels so good.
Monique, 18 – Ashley, 5 months

Children Need to Be Active

Physical activity is important for all of us. This includes your infant. Give him plenty of chances to be active. He needs room to move around. Let him crawl all over you. He'll be learning to coordinate his body movements as he crawls.

Crawl around with him while you play peek-a-boo and hide-and-go-seek. As he's beginning to crawl, place a toy he likes across the room from him. Does he go after it? He might enjoy playing a grab-the-toy game as you move it all around the room for him.

As he begins to walk, play games with him. Chase him around the room and across the yard. Make healthy activity more fun than watching TV.

Children become healthier and stronger if they get large muscle exercise every day. Doing exercises indoors can help, too. Choose children's TV that includes dancing, jumping, or other exercise. Limit all other TV or computer time.

Play music that makes everyone want to move. Dance or march around the house. Sing and make the experience fun.

When you're in a safe space, take your child out of his stroller and let him walk beside you. It may take longer, but it is a wonderful experience for your child.

Can you walk to the neighborhood store or preschool with your child? At the mall, take the stairs instead of the elevator or escalator. Let him help you when you're working outside.

If you have an older child, talk to him about how he wants to exercise each day.

> *I do worry about her weight. Since she started crawling, she actually has lost a couple of ounces. She's not burning it off as quick since she's starting to walk. When she gets older we'll worry about going for walks, stuff like that.*
>
> Ameera

Weight loss and improved health can be accomplished with only 30-60 minutes of walking each day. Everything counts. Break the time into several small walks, and before you know it, you'll be feeling better.

The Fat and Sugar Jungle

> *I know a bunch of people who eat Cheetos® and drink Mountain Dew® all the time. Their babies are going to come out crazy, hyperactive.*
>
> *My one friend is eight months pregnant with twin boys. She won't eat any fruit or any vegetables. She drinks juice once in awhile, and eats a lot of meat, but she also eats a lot of chips and ice cream.*
>
> Chika, 16 – 4 months pregnant

Now to step two. Look at what you eat and how it matches the recommendations in Chapter 1 and MyPyramid,
pp. 49-50. The best way to learn more about MyPyramid is
to go to **<www.mypyramid.gov>** It provides advice based
on your age, size, and activity level. You can even enter
your favorite foods or those you prefer not to eat.

Now the questions are:

* How does this match what you eat now?

* How does it apply to what you give your child to eat?

* How does your weight and your child's weight fit with
  the recommendations for your height and his age?

* Has your health care professional suggested that you
  should weigh less?

* What about your child?

*I don't like to give Julian candy or cookies. Some
people give him a sucker and I don't like it. I don't
want him to get into the habit of eating suckers or
other sweet things.*

Cynthia, 17 – Julian, 11 months

Even if you think he's overweight, don't put your child
on a restrictive diet. Instead, think of lots of ways to shift
from high-fat, high-sugar snacks to foods with fewer calories. Offer fruit, yogurt, or carrot sticks as a snack. If he's
already learned to want candy and cookies every day, don't
expect him to stop all at once. Encourage him to eat smaller
portions, and offer this kind of food less often.

Throw Out Junk Food

The best thing is to get those high-calorie unhealthy
foods out of your house. Quit buying sodas. Bake or buy
cookies less often. Let dessert be fruit. Save the rich cake
for special occasions.

Your child may like the juice drinks or blends that come in boxes or pouches. These have very little juice and are more expensive than plain juice. They also contain a lot of sugar. Again, you're paying a lot for water, sugar, and packaging.

Juice doesn't have to be in a box. There are many special cups for children, and they're washable. So you save money there, too.

Most of us think of fruit juice as being nutritious. Children like it because it's sweet, tastes good, and is conveniently packaged. Like soda and fruit drinks, however, fruit juice can be one cause of weight gain.

A study of children aged two to five years showed that those who drank 12 ounces or more of fruit juice daily were more likely to be obese. Whole fruit is a better choice because of the fiber it contains.

Stock up on nutritious foods. Keep a bowl of fruit on the counter where your child can help himself. Pretzels are another reasonable snack. (See page 178 for a recipe for pretzels that your child can help you make.)

Perhaps you'll decide on a new rule — no eating in front of the TV. (It's too easy to snack endlessly once you've started and you're absorbed in a show.)

Do you cook most of your meals at home? Avoiding fast foods, vending machines, and highly processed foods is important because most of these foods are high in calories and low in nutrition.

Your parents probably said many times to you, "Eat your vegetables. No dessert until you do." A better way with your child is to make dessert also a healthy choice. Offer good foods, but your child decides what he will eat.

Other steps to help prevent a weight problem for your child:

- Don't offer food as a reward. A hug is better.

• You can't expect a toddler to change food habits
  overnight. Make changes gradually.

Are All Carbohydrates Bad?

A popular weight-reducing diet is extremely low in
carbohydrates. Some people have tried to lose weight by
seriously cutting back on the carbohydrates they eat. They
may eat far fewer carbohydrates than recommended for
healthy living.

This is not good because we need a reasonable amount of
healthy carbohydrates in our diet each day.

So what's wrong with sugar? Sugar, along with starch, is
a carbohydrate. The three nutrients that provide calories and
give us energy are carbohydrates, protein, and fat. We need
all three of these nutrients plus vitamins and minerals for
energy, growth, and good health.

As you know, good sources of carbohydrates include

• whole grain cereals

• brown rice

• whole grain breads

• fruits

• vegetables

However, meeting our daily need for carbohydrates
through soft drinks, candy, and other high-sugar foods with
little or no other nutrients does nothing good for our bodies.
If we rely on these foods for our carbohydrate needs, we
can't possibly get the nutrients so essential for our health
and our family's health.

> At school I notice they tend to snack on the wrong
> things. Like potato chips, but I can kind of understand
> that . . . I try not to eat junk food – like some of the
> girls are using pregnancy as an excuse to eat. They

*say they're craving a bag of potato chips, so that's
what they eat.*

Nhu, 17 – almost 9 months pregnant

The Sugar Monster

*When Luis was about 3 years old, he had big cavi-
ties, and I had to take him to the children's hospital
for dental surgery. I hate going to the dentist and I
know how he felt, so now I limit all that sweet stuff.
Instead of straight juice, I dilute it.*

*I changed a lot when he went to the dentist. It
broke my heart, all that dental work. Everything that
happens to him now is because of me.*

*I limit the fast foods and the kinds of snacks. Before
I would just give him Snickers® or whatever. Now it's
things like yogurt and granola or chopped fruit
and yogurt.*

Carlota, 18 – Luis, 4 1/2

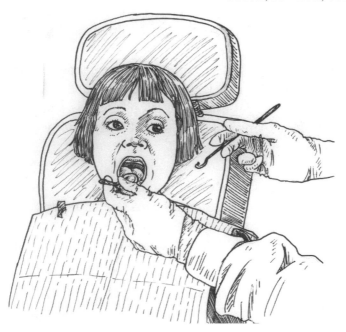

Carlota and Luis learned the hard way that too much sugar often leads to cavities. And cavities mean trips to the dentist.

There are several ways to help your child avoid those painful cavities.

- First, cut back on the amount of sugar she eats.
- Cut back on the *number of times* she eats sugary foods. Each time she eats sugar, acid forms on her teeth. The damage occurs within the first 15-20 minutes after she eats the sugar.
- Insist that your child brush her teeth or rinse out her mouth right after eating foods containing sugar.

Do most of us eat more sugar than we need? Let's start by looking at some facts.

Did you know that a 12-ounce can of soda contains 9 teaspoons of sugar? That's 3 tablespoons. One of the fast food places recently advertised a 64-ounce drink for 64¢. That would be a full cup of sugar. A cup of sugar contains 720 calories.

If you're an average American, you're eating about 130 pounds of sugar a year. That's about 1/3 pound a day, or 2/3 cup (480 calories). While some people eat less and some more, health experts tell us we could all benefit by eating less sugar.

Sugar Equals Calories

We know that eating sugar means taking in more calories — 45 calories per tablespoon of sugar. Too many calories and too little exercise result in stored fat in our bodies.

I try not to give Jabari a lot of sweets, but my mom does. Every time he sees her, he wants a piece of candy.

I tell her I don't want him to have it, and she says,
"He can just taste it."

Abeni, 17 – Jabari, 16 months; Abiba, 6 weeks

A national report of the Feeding Infants and Toddlers
study showed that one in four infants 6-12 months old
exceeded mean energy intake. That is, they ate more than
they needed.

About half of babies aged 7 to 8 months eat some kind of
dessert or sweet beverages. This percentage goes up as they
grow older. Young children do not need sweet beverages.
Save sweet, fat-laden desserts for an occasional treat.

Eating these foods means baby doesn't have room for the
healthy foods she needs. This is something you may need to
explain to other people who are convinced a cookie is equal
to love. Babies and children who don't get the nutrients in
healthy foods can't behave as well or learn as well as they
should. It isn't "love" to make life harder for them.

Johnnie's mom and dad wanted to give Danté
cookies at two months! That frustrated me because
I knew he shouldn't have it. When they'd hold him,
they'd give him the cookie. Then I'd take him and take
the cookie away.

Argentina

Beverages May Be a Problem

A big source of sugar for any child is the drinks they're
offered. Few beverages other than breast milk, milk, and
pure fruit juices have significant food value.

It's best to introduce your child to drinking water when
he first begins drinking from a cup. But if that hasn't
happened, it's *not* too late to change.

Begin by thinking about what you drink. If you guzzle
soda all day, why wouldn't your child want the same thing?
Maybe you'll think about yourself and the empty calories

you're getting. And if you drink diet sodas, you're spending a lot of money for flavored water.

If you're drinking lots of soda, how do you think you could cut back? Caimile probably had a much bigger challenge than you'll ever have — she was drinking 12 cans of soda a day! Then, because of her pregnancy, her doctor asked her to stop completely:

> *I used to drink a 12-pack of Dr. Pepper® every day. I constantly had a pop in my hands. Then, while I was pregnant, I had to cut out caffeine.*
>
> *I read about how women stop smoking, and how you can wean yourself. So I applied that to pop. The first week I drank the same. The second week, I cut back by one, with 11 cans a day. I did this for several weeks, and by 5 months, I had cut pop out completely.*
>
> *I felt tired, either because of caffeine or the pregnancy, but I felt better after I stopped.*
>
> Caimile, 17 – Hajari, 4 months

If your child drinks one 12-ounce can of sweetened soft drink each day, her risk of becoming obese is increased.

At home, offer water when your child says he's thirsty. Remember that sugared drinks not only raise the blood sugar levels, they also cause serious tooth decay.

> *At 4 months, Johnny's sister wanted to give Danté diluted Kool-Aid® in a bottle. I had to be a little forceful. When she'd start giving him Kool-Aid® I'd go over and start playing with him, then say, "He's ready to eat."*
>
> *At first, Johnny agreed with his parents. He'd say, "Well, they never get to see him, and they want to hold him." I said Danté was too young to have Kool-Aid®. Then Johnny started agreeing with me.*
>
> Argentina

Instead of Kool-Aid® type drinks, try mixing plain juice with water. Just fill the cup 1/4 full of juice, then fill with water. Let your child color his water/water-juice mixture with food coloring. It also gives you a chance to talk about color names and make fun combinations, such as red and yellow for orange or red and blue for purple.

Managing Eating Out

One of the greatest challenges to healthy eating is eating away from home. In fast food restaurants it is especially difficult to make good eating choices because most foods served there are more than 30 percent fat. (See chapter 4.)

The sights and smells of the foods around you are tempting. Even if you're careful, it's hard to find much variety in healthy choices.

At some restaurants, even the choices of simple foods such as chicken or a salad may be bad. Often these dishes are fried, covered with sauces, or have high fat dressings.

When low-fat choices are offered, get in the habit of making that choice. Many restaurants now mark the things that are "heart healthy" with a star or special mark. This lets you know they are low in fat and sugar. Enjoy them!

Maybe people in your family have a hard time keeping their weight within a normal range. Various genetic differences cause some families to gain weight easily and some to struggle to keep their weight high enough. Other families don't seem to have to think about weight at all.

Whatever the case in your family, know that eating well (eating the healthy foods you need) makes a more satisfying life for you and your child. *What you eat matters!*

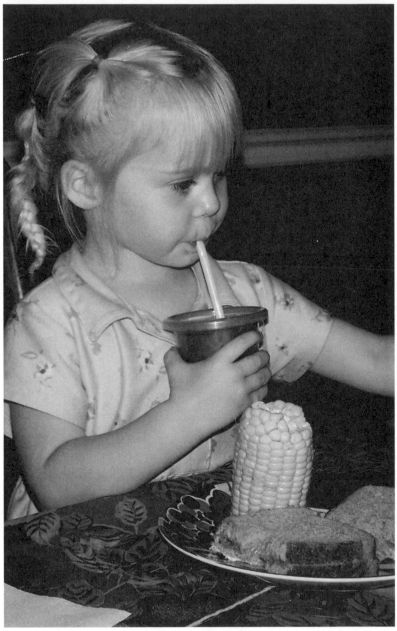

Perhaps she'd also like a dark green vegetable or carrot sticks along with her corn and peanut butter sandwich.

8

Extra Planning for Vegetarian Kids

- **Good Food for Vegetarians**

- **Pregnancy and Vegetarianism**

- **Special Vegetarian Choices**

- **While You're Breastfeeding**

- **Feeding Your Vegetarian Baby**

- **Vegetarian Diet for Toddlers**

- **Preschooler's Nutrient Needs Expand**

- **Plan, Plan, Plan!**

I'm a vegetarian and Lamont will be, too. I still breastfeed, pretty much just at night. I never used any bottles. I did this because I wanted him to be as healthy as possible.

At about five months, I started giving him solid food. The first thing was a banana in a jar but he didn't like it. I tried it, and I couldn't believe they called that bananas. So I gave him applesauce. Later I mashed a real banana and he liked it.

Pretty soon I started giving him rice cereal.

Delila, 17 – Lamont, 14 months

Good Food for Vegetarians

Are you or your family vegetarian? That is, do you choose not to eat meat, poultry or fish? Some people are even stricter about not eating animal products. They don't eat eggs or milk, and they're called vegans.

Vegetarianism can be a healthy way to go, even during pregnancy, breastfeeding, and for small children. To be healthy, however, means your diet and your child's diet must be well balanced. It's even more important that vegetarians eat a wide variety of food including greens, fruits and vegetables, beans, nuts or seeds, eggs and dairy products (unless they're vegan), and a small amount of fat.

Please see MyPyramid on pp. 49-50. If you go to the website (**<mypyramid.gov>**), you can find "Tips and Resources for Vegetarian Diets."

Whole grains and legumes (soy, beans, peanuts, and others) are especially important for vegetarians as are fruits and vegetables. If you're vegetarian, you need to eat some of each of these foods — whole grains, legumes, fruits and vegetables — at every meal.

Each day, a vegetarian should have some nuts or seeds, plant oils, eggs, dairy foods, and/or soymilk plus vegetables and fruits. Each of the groups provides some, but not all, of the nutrients you need. Don't try to replace foods in one group with foods in another. It won't work nutritionally. All these food groups are important. For good health, you and your child need them all.

Pregnancy and Vegetarianism

During pregnancy I ate lots of cheese. I don't like milk, so I usually have it with cereal or if I'm eating something really sweet. I eat cottage cheese, yogurt, and I take vitamins.

Delila

You already know how much protein is needed during pregnancy — 50-70 grams daily. It supports the rapid growth of the fetus and placenta and also the growth of maternal tissue. You consume about ten grams of protein each time you eat or drink any one of the following:

- 1 1/2 cups soymilk
- 3 1/2 ounces extra-firm tofu
- 3 ounces tempeh (cultured soybeans with a chewy texture)
- 1 large whole-grain bagel
- 1/2 cup cooked beans
- 2 tablespoons peanut butter

You need iron during pregnancy because of the increase in blood in your body and the blood forming for your fetus. Choose such iron-rich foods as:

- whole grains
- legumes
- tofu
- dark green leafy vegetables

When you eat these foods along with food rich in vitamin C, your body will absorb more of the iron. Taking an iron supplement, especially during your second and third trimesters, would be wise. Check with your healthcare provider.

Getting plenty of calcium is also especially important during pregnancy because it helps build your baby's bones and teeth. If you eat dairy products, you should get enough calcium from four or five cups of milk and a serving of cheese.

A pregnant vegetarian, just like other pregnant women, only needs 300-400 extra calories a day, an increase of about 18 percent. At the same time, her nutrient needs increase about 50 percent. Obviously vegetarian women need to choose foods especially rich in nutrients. Just like non-vegetarians, they should eat very little candy and other sweets.

If you're either vegan or lactose-intolerant (you can't drink milk), you need to plan how you'll still get plenty of calcium. Some brands of soy and rice milk, fruit juices, cereals and waffles are fortified with calcium. Soybeans, dark green leafy vegetables like collard greens, kale, broccoli, and turnip greens, and tofu are other sources of calcium.

Soymilk or rice milk costs a little more, but either of these choices provide almost as much calcium and other important nutrients as cow's milk does.

> *We drink rice or soymilk. I'm lactose intolerant. Cheese and yogurt are not a problem.*
>
> *My boyfriend thought this would be a big change — having different milk in the refrigerator. It does taste different, and I prefer the chocolate. He thought it was going to be this big thing to change over, but it took him maybe a week to get used to it. That's what we have now.*
>
> Hannah, 23 – Mackenzie, 41/2

Dietary Guidelines for Americans state that those who eat only plant foods must supplement their diet with vitamins B_{12}, vitamin D, calcium, iron, and zinc. This is even more important for growing children and pregnant and lactating women. Check with your doctor or pharmacist.

Special Vegetarian Choices

Many foods that usually include meat or poultry can be adapted to vegetarian eating. Some examples from MyPyramid:

- pasta primavera or pasta with marinara or pesto sauce
- veggie pizza
- vegetable lasagna
- tofu-vegetable stir fry
- vegetable lo mein
- vegetable kabobs
- bean burritos or tacos

You can find a variety of vegetarian products that look, and may even taste like their non-vegetarian counterparts. These are usually lower in saturated fat and contain no cholesterol.

Soy-based sausage patties or links taste good with eggs at breakfast. Veggie burgers are a good-tasting substitute for hamburgers. You can find veggie burgers made with soy beans, vegetables, and/or rice.

You can add tempeh, tofu, or wheat gluten (seitan) to soups and stews. This adds protein without saturated fat or cholesterol.

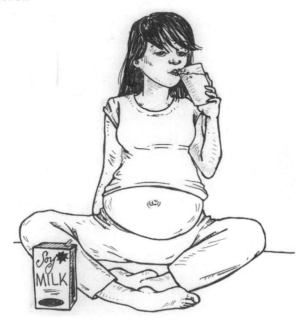

Have you eaten falafel (spicy ground chick peas)? You can use this to make bean burgers, lentil burgers, or to fill pita halves.

Many Asian and Indian restaurants offer a varied selection of vegetarian dishes.

If you're underweight, or you're having a hard time eating enough food to meet the needs of you and your baby, choose nutritious foods higher in calories. (Vegetarians are more likely than non-vegetarians to consume fewer calories than they need.)

If you need more calories rich in nutrients, you might like milkshakes made of soymilk or cow's milk blended with fruit and tofu or yogurt. Other possibilities include eating more nuts and nut butter such as peanut or almond butter, dried fruits, soy products and bean dips. If you find it hard to eat enough at meals, try to eat more often.

While You're Breastfeeding

You don't need to drink cow's milk to make milk for your baby, but as a vegetarian or vegan you have about the same nutrient needs as other breastfeeding mothers. You will simply choose different foods.

You need about 500 extra calories daily when you're breastfeeding, You need even more calcium than you did while you were pregnant. If you don't drink milk, include an extra portion of calcium-rich food in your diet:

- calcium-fortified tofu
- bok choy, broccoli, other dark green leafy vegetables
- calcium-fortified soymilk
- calcium-fortified rice milk
- calcium-fortified cereals

As mentioned before, make sure you're getting enough

vitamins D and B$_{12}$, probably through a supplement. You'll also get some vitamin B$_{12}$ in fortified cereal and soymilk, but it's not in most plant foods.

Fifteen minutes of sun each day provides enough vitamin D. Use sunscreen after fifteen minutes.

As you breastfeed, you need even more protein than you did during pregnancy, about five additional grams. Carefully selected plant-based foods and soy protein are good sources.

Feeding Your Vegetarian Baby

Vegetarian babies, like all babies, do best on breast milk the first six months. Those who are bottle-fed need nothing except formula.

By six months, gradually introduce other foods to your baby. See chapter 3 for detailed information. From six to nine or ten months, a vegetarian baby's diet is likely to be the same as recommended for all babies in this chapter.

By ten months, baby's food can be chopped, finely grated, or blended. If you've checked carefully for allergies, and he appears not to have this problem, you can start combination foods. Blending avocado and tofu or applesauce or cooked greens with peanut butter may appeal to him, for example. (But be sure he's not allergic to peanuts.)

At first he would eat almost everything, and then he started not eating any green foods like peas or broccoli. So the only way he would eat it would be having it mixed with something else, like peas and brown rice. Then he started finger foods, and he didn't want to be fed out of the jar.

He got real picky. I would give him the same thing as I had, but he would throw it off his tray and grab it off my plate. For some reason he thought my food would be better.

Now he likes lots of cheese. Everything has cheese

in it. He still doesn't like broccoli, but he will eat it
mixed with macaroni and cheese. I also mix green
beans or peas with macaroni and cheese.

Delila

Tasting a wide variety of vegetables and fruits is even
more important for a vegan or vegetarian baby. By now, he
can eat spinach and cabbage along with root vegetables.
He's ready for well-cooked whole grains, and also for
high-protein cereals such as soybeans and wheat germ.

Vegetarian Diet for Toddlers

He likes to eat pizza (more cheese). He likes pasta,
bread. I really like grilled peanut butter and jelly
sandwiches and he loves those. He likes to snack on
crackers with cheese or peanut butter on them. If I
have a bean burrito he will eat part of mine.

He has a lot of dairy products, scrambled eggs.
One meal he really likes — I fry some corn tortillas
(cut in triangles), scramble some eggs with them, then
melt cheese on it. Then I add cut-up tomatoes and
avocados.

He has eggs at least three times a week. Cheese
every day. Cheese on crackers, vegetables, toast and
cheese. It's usually Cheddar or Monterey jack. His
favorite is Cheddar. He drinks milk better when he's
in daycare. They say when they're around their mom
they want the breast milk.

Delila

Adult vegetarian diets are usually low in fat and high in
fiber. Infants and all children under five years can feel full
on this diet before they've eaten food with adequate energy
(calories) and nutrition. Because of this fact, vegetarian
diets for infants and small children need to include fewer

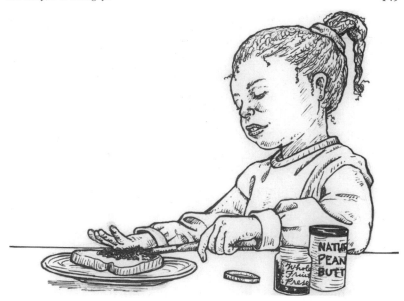

high-fiber foods and more energy and nutrient-dense foods than adults need.

This does not mean filling your vegetarian child up with French fries and soda!

Your one-year-old can eat the same meals as the rest of the family. She will also need snacks between meals. Include dried peas and beans in her menu, but be sure they are cooked quite soft. Skins, especially on soya, should be removed before serving to a one-year-old.

Try a thin split-pea soup as an introduction to legume protein. You can see if the peas and beans are being digested well by checking your child's stool. If the stool smells sour, or baby's bottom is red or irritated, or if you can still see parts of the beans, wait awhile before trying legumes again.

Some children can't handle whole legumes until they are two, or even three years old. If this is the case with your child, meet her nutrition needs with other soy products such as soymilk, tofu, and greens.

Hummus, made with chickpeas and tahini (sesame seed

butter) contains lots of protein and calcium. Your child is
likely to enjoy eating it. See the Quick Crispy Snack recipe
on p. 178 (toasted pita bread and hummus).

Avocado is a great food for babies. It's rich in ribofla-
vin, essential fatty acids, potassium, and copper. Let her eat
small pieces with her fingers.

Most small children like noodles. Get pasta enriched
with spinach or other vegetable flours. You provide your
child with energy and protein when you serve it.

By now, your child can enjoy raw vegetables, such as
carrots and cucumbers, if they are finely grated. Of course
you wouldn't offer her a carrot stick at one year of age
because of the choking danger.

Preschooler's Nutrient Needs Expand

*Mackenzie eats a lot of peanut butter. She usually
has two pieces of peanut butter toast and a banana
for breakfast every morning. She loves peanut butter
sandwiches.*

She also takes a vitamin every day.

Hannah, 23 - Mackenzie, 41/2

Review chapter 6 for suggestions on feeding preschoolers who are not vegetarian. Your vegetarian preschooler
needs the same nutrients as other children, but will get them
from greens, legumes, fruits and vegetables, nuts and seeds,
soymilk, and, if he is not vegan, milk and eggs.

Plant protein can provide enough protein if the individual eats a variety of plant foods. However, some experts
say that, based on the lower digestibility of plant proteins,
vegetarian babies up to age 2 may need 30-35 percent more
protein than non-vegetarians. Vegetarian children aged two
to six years old may need 20-30 percent more plant proteins.

The quality of plant protein varies. Isolated soy protein

can meet protein needs as well as animal protein. Wheat protein, when eaten alone, may be 50 percent less usable by the body than protein from animals.

To get enough protein on a vegetarian diet, you and your child need to consume a wide variety of plant protein foods. Eaten alone, some of this protein is incomplete. Frequent meals and snacks plus some refined foods (such as fortified breakfast cereals, breads, and pasta) can help vegetarian children meet their energy and nutrient needs.

Seeds, such as sunflower and pumpkin, make good snacks. (See recipe for pumpkin seeds on p. 179.) Almond butter on a slice of bread provides protein.

Other snack possibilities include raisins, prunes, carrot sticks (after age 3), hard-boiled eggs, and cheese sticks.

Plan, Plan, Plan!

Planning a good-tasting and healthy vegetarian diet is much like planning any healthy diet. Include a variety of foods from each of the food groups. Be aware of possible nutrient deficiencies in your child's diet and figure out how you will see that she gets those nutrients.

Choose whole, unrefined foods often. Eat very little highly sweetened, fatty and heavily refined foods. Choose a wide variety of fruits and vegetables.

A vegetarian diet can be a healthy choice for your child and for you. But it must be planned. It's a good idea to get some professional help. Talk to your family healthcare provider, pediatrician, or a registered dietician.

Search for "vegetarian" on the Internet and you'll find help. Also consult good vegetarian cookbooks.

Both you and your child need to eat food containing adequate nutrients. As you plan, you will undoubtedly find more vegetarian choices than you realized existed.

You and your child will benefit from your planning.

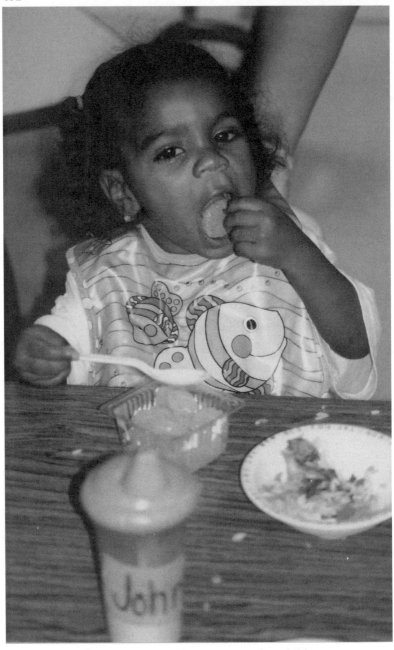

She's getting good food and loving care at her childcare center.

9

Good Food and Childcare

They have to offer rice cereal until he's a year old. They give him that and some peaches or other fruit at breakfast. For lunch, chicken and rice, peas, and mandarin oranges.

I'm 20 miles away from my school, and the only reason I go there is the daycare and the GRADS program. There are usually about eight children with four people to take care of them.

Cynthia, 17 – Julian, 11 months

Felicia goes to a private home for daycare, one with 9-14 children. They give them

*carrots, cheese, salad, crackers, sandwiches. The
other day it was barbequed chicken, salad, and
strawberries.*

*The kids serve themselves. It's real cute. They teach
them to hold their cups with both hands.*

*The food there seems to be very good, and not
candy and pizza.*

Kristi Ann, 18 – Felicia, 2½

Childcare Settings Vary

Many children in young families spend time in childcare
settings. These are often wonderful places for a child to be
while parents are at work or school.

You can find many helpful materials to assist you in making a good selection of care that best matches your child. It
may be in a home setting with a family member or friend. It
could be a licensed in-home childcare location.

In many school locations childcare is available on or near
the school campus. If it's at your school, this may be what
you and your child need.

*Moises goes to daycare at school. They feed him
stuff like burritos or pizza. I'm not too big on these
foods. This isn't too often, but if I were going to worry,
it would be the burritos and pizza.*

*They also do stuff like chicken and pasta, and that's
what I like him to eat.*

Melinda Jane, 16 – Moises, 15 months

Most group childcare centers have guidelines they must
follow for feeding young children. Those guidelines come
from various sources such as Departments of Education,
WIC, Head Start, Early Head Start, and State licensing
agencies. However, not all guidelines are alike. If you move
from one kind of care to another, the food given to your
child may change a little, too.

*Zaila is in Head Start. They have to have one serv-
ing from each food group in each meal. Today they
had chopped beef nuggets, broccoli, applesauce,
dinner roll, whole milk, and strawberry bites. For
breakfast they usually have cereal, milk, and orange
juice. They post preferences of the various children.*

Jasmine, 19 – Zaila, 3; Cody, 7 months

Ask Lots of Questions

It's important to visit any site with which you aren't
familiar. For example, a friend visited a childcare center one
morning. The children were having breakfast — but they
weren't much interested in eating. There they were, six toddlers in high chairs, lined up against a wall, watching TV,
with a bowl of dry, sugary cereal on each high chair tray.
That's *not* what you want for your child.

Toddlers don't need sugar-filled cereal. They don't need
TV while they eat. And they certainly do need friendly at-
tention during meals, whether that attention comes from
Mom or Dad, or from another caregiver.

Even with a family member or friend, it's important to
make your wishes for your child's care known from the
beginning. You need to ask about the usual practices for
serving food while your child is there.

Your questions might include:

• Do you provide breakfast? If so, what do you serve?
  Are those things your child usually eats? If not, ask
  how they handle offering new foods to your child. If it
  seems advisable, can you bring his meals?

*Sometimes she doesn't eat as good as she should
there. They don't have enough vegetables and fruits.
Sometimes they give them French toast for lunch, and
I think they need something healthier than that.*

Kaitlyn, 16 – Madison, 2

- When are snacks offered? What are the usual snacks? Are juices diluted with water? Remember, the whole fruit is better for your child than too much juice. Four to six ounces of juice a day is plenty for a preschooler. A toddler needs less. Is just water offered as a choice?

- What time is lunch served? What is the usual menu? How do you handle a child's varying hunger? Do you insist on "clean plates"?

- If your child has any allergies, ask how they make certain that she will not be given a food she cannot eat.

- If your child takes a bottle, will they always hold him at each feeding? (No propped bottles!) How do they help a child learn to drink from a cup?

- If a child says she is hungry at a time other than a regular meal or snack time, what happens? Usually, however, children don't say they're hungry. Instead, they start being fussy or acting out. Frequent healthy snacks are essential.

In private care such as with relatives or friends, asking about these things may be a little touchy. Spend some time

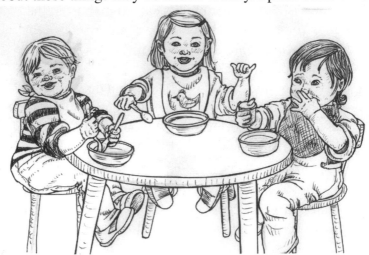

at the place your child will be. Observe how feeding and various discipline issues are handled. How well do they match what you want your child to experience? For example, is eating a certain food tied to "dessert"?

What If He Doesn't Eat?

Remember the ten-tries rule. Ask the child to taste a tiny bite of the new food. If he doesn't think he wants any more, that's okay. But keep offering a bite each time that food is served. It may take ten or fifteen tries before he decides it's good.

Does the caregiver share your feeling about this? If the child doesn't want to eat, what happens? In many families there are strong feelings about this and other practices related to food. It will save a lot of difficulty later if the caregiver's practices pretty well match your own.

Individual families as well as ethnic groups often prefer specific foods. Will your child find familiar dishes at childcare, at least part of the time?

Can you pack a lunch for your child to take with him?

When first separated from their mothers, many children are not able to eat much in the new place. The food should be offered but the child's response should be respected. As children begin to feel at home in the new environment, their appetite increases and they return to their former eating habits.

> *During lunch I go down to daycare with Jamie.*
> *They use Hamburger Helper® which has preserva-*
> *tives in it. They eat what's convenient, but they offer a*
> *variety, and do pretty good.*
>
> Monique, 18 – Ashley, 5 months

Are you able to visit your preschooler at mealtime during the first few days? That could help him adjust more quickly.

Younger children may do better telling Mom goodbye only once.

You may choose or be asked to take treats occasionally for the children at your child's center, perhaps to celebrate a birthday or other holiday. Remember that a "treat" does not have to be a cupcake with thick icing served with a sugary fruit drink.

Most children would enjoy cut-up melon and other kinds of fruit plus fruit juice diluted with water. On St. Patrick's Day, perhaps they'd be intrigued with green milk and green sugar-free jello with fruit in it. Use your imagination.

Communication Is Crucial

How do your child's caregivers communicate with you? You need to be told about anything unusual that has happened. They also need to discuss with you any special needs your child may have had during the day.

Ideally, you'll be told how well the child eats each day. They will probably also discuss with you how active your child was throughout the day and how much he participated in the various activities.

> *The people at daycare give me a list of what Jabari eats during the day. They know his favorite foods are bananas and peaches, but I've never seen him turn something down.*
> Abeni, 17 – Jabari, 16 months; Abiba, 6 weeks

If communication between you and your child's caregiver(s) is incomplete, you need to find a way to talk together on a regular basis. You may need to request a specific time when you can talk.

Childcare at School

Talk with your child's caregiver about how you want to provide healthy food for your child. Ideally, the caregiver will join you in teaching your child about nutrition and the foods he should eat each day.

Becky Escoto, head teacher at Artesia Children's Center, ABCUSD, Artesia, CA, works hard to encourage better eating among the children. "When a child talks about buying soda when they get their hamburger, we say, 'No, no soda with your hamburger. Ask Mom to buy you milk together with your hamburger.'

"We ask, 'What did you do this weekend?'

"'Oh, we went to Chuck E. Cheese®.'

"'Did you buy soda or did you get milk?' Some say soda, some say milk.

"Once in awhile a parent says, 'Becky, they told me they had to order milk. They shouldn't get soda.'

"'Oh, yes,' I reply. Parents are seldom upset."

Becky discussed their nutrition curriculum at the Center.

"In our lessons we do health and foods, a little of MyPyramid. One month we may do something on vegetables and fruits. Another time we'll incorporate another part of MyPyramid. And of course we have discussions. What is good food? What is bad food?"

We asked Becky if the kids eat what they serve. She said, "The macaroni and cheese go quickly, and so does the burrito. When we have rice and an egg roll, some of them don't eat it, but others love it. They all drink milk, although some are on soymilk and Lactaid® plus 2 percent regular milk.

"Here they have to have a balanced meal, which the district provides. They often have salad or a fruit cup with milk. They eat carrots with salad dressing," Becky concluded.

Caregivers who attend to young children are generally experienced and devoted to the good care children deserve.

Let your child's caregiver join with you in making your child's days in childcare a happy, healthy experience for both of you.

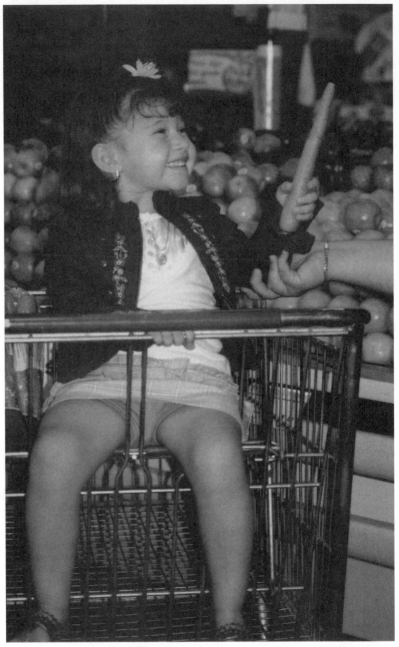

She's having a great time helping Mom do the weekly shopping.

10

Food Shopping and Your Budget

- **Cook and Save**
- **Three-Generation Living**
- **Planning Your Shopping**
- **Coupons Can Help**
- **Buying Fresh Produce**
- **Tips for Buying Meat**
- **Pork, Poultry and Fish**
- **Two-Family Households**
- **Your Toddler Can Help**

Buy only food you know you're going to cook. Use the foods in different ways. Learn about nutrition if you want to have strong kids.

I don't buy prepared food. I think it's nasty.

Chloe, 22 – Alyssa, 2; Denae, 1

I have to watch my spending a lot. Going from me working, both of us, then me quitting was a huge change.

We don't have to buy the juice boxes or the prepared snack foods.

I think junk food costs so much.

We used to drink a lot of soda. We added it up one day — look how much money we're spending buying all this soda. It was kind of a gradual thing, a money thing. "Look how much we can save," and we quit.

Hannah, 23 – Mackenzie, 4 1/2

Cook and Save

Healthy, nutritious food can be expensive. Preparing it at home takes time. It's easy to understand why many people think going to a restaurant or a fast-food place is good for many of their meals.

Of course eating out is almost always more expensive.

When I lived with my mom before the first pregnancy, my mom cooked and we didn't eat out a lot. When I moved out I was lazy. It was easier to get a pizza or go to McDonald's®. But when you think about it, you can buy a week's groceries for about the price of a visit to McDonald's®.

Ukari, 19 – Kendall, 3

Serving TV dinners and other already-prepared foods at home almost always provides less food, and certainly less nutritious dishes, for your money than do foods you make "from scratch."

Time and money spent on groceries and preparing and cooking your own food is well spent. You can fix a more nutritious and appetizing meal. It may not even take more time if you add up the time spent traveling to and from the restaurant, ordering your food, and waiting to be served.

Three-Generation Living

Perhaps you live with your parents or your partner's parents. You may feel you don't have a lot to do with the food choices in your home. If this is the case, you may want to offer to help more with the meal planning, food shopping, and food preparation. If you do, you may have more opportunity to influence your child's eating, as well as your own.

You're probably very busy most days. So look for simply prepared foods, menus you can fix in the short time you have. Well-planned, simple meals can be just as delicious and sometimes more healthy than dishes that take lots of time and effort to prepare.

Those simple meals can definitely be healthier and as tasty as using already-prepared foods from the supermarket. You'll also save money by preparing the food yourself.

Planning Your Shopping

So how do you shop for food without going bankrupt in the process? First, buy only what you need. To do this, keep a shopping list in a place where you and others can write down items you need.

It also helps to plan your meals, at least the main dishes, for the week. If you live with your parents, they might appreciate some help with this task. Think about which days you may have time to cook and which days everyone will be rushed. Figure out how to serve healthy foods you can afford without spending more time than you have. Now there's a challenge!

Plan your food shopping trip before you leave home. Check out the food ads for several stores close enough for you to visit. Choose the store that has specials that best fit your needs.

If you can get to a supermarket, it's more economical to shop there than at a convenience store. Convenience stores tend to be what they say they are — convenient. Along with the convenience, you'll probably pay more for most items. You may also find a poor selection of foods, and the food may not be as fresh as you find in many supermarkets.

Make sure you aren't hungry when you shop. If you are,

you're much more likely to buy things that look good but you don't really need.

When you go in the store, pick up the newspaper/advertising flyer the store publishes. Scan the ads. You may find something on sale that fits into your eating plan. If the sale item is not perishable, you can buy it now and fit it into your next food plan.

Do you have a calculator? You might want to take it along with you so you can add up costs as you shop. You'll be less likely to go over your food budget.

Remember, for the price of a large bag of chips and a box of cookies, you could buy lots of fruits and vegetables. When you get home, make those fruits and vegetables handy for snacking. Perhaps you'll prepare baggies with raisins or raw vegetables for your preschooler's snacks.

Coupons Can Help

Are you a coupon clipper? You can save money by using coupons. However, don't buy something only because you have a coupon that makes it cheaper — be sure you buy only what you need.

The key to using coupons effectively is in organizing them. Perhaps you'll have an envelope for each kind of food — canned food, baby food, cereal and breads, fresh food, frozen items, cleaning supplies, etc.

After you've clipped coupons from the Sunday paper, Internet, or mail, plan your menus for the next week. If you at least have a basic plan for meals, your shopping will go better. You're more likely to buy only what you need rather than doing impulse shopping.

I use the Club card at Vons®, so it's kind of like coupons. I think it depends on where you go, whether or not you clip coupons.

Ukari

If your supermarket has its own shopping card, remember to use it. It generally allows a discount on some of the items you need.

Many things found in the grocery stores come with some packages having name brands and some with store brand labels. The store's own brand of foods will usually be cheaper than the big-name brands. Generally the products inside are very much alike. Since the store brand is usually much cheaper, there is little reason to buy the name brand. In fact, sometimes the store brand may be packaged at the same place as the name brand.

Most canned and packaged foods will have a price per unit tag on the shelf it's setting on. When you see several brands of an item you need, whether it's food, cleaning supplies, toilet paper, or something else, read the price per unit. Prices often vary significantly among the different brands. For example, it might be 7¢ an ounce for one brand versus 19¢ an ounce on another. It pays to be alert to these little signs. Usually the higher priced brands are placed at eye level. If you have to stretch or stoop to reach items, they

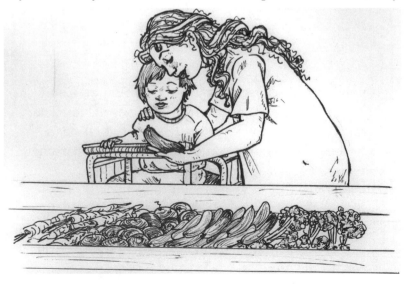

may be cheaper.

It's best to complete your shopping before you reach the cash register. It's usually surrounded with impulse items that look inviting but you may not need.

Buying Fresh Produce

If you read the ads, you'll find certain vegetables and fruits are featured, usually those in season. It's wise to choose these foods because they're probably cheaper. This also means more people are buying them, so the turnover is higher. This translates to fresher fruits and vegetables.

It's best to buy fruits and vegetables to last about a week. You'll get more vitamins if you eat fruits and vegetables while they're fresh. They'll also taste better.

Frozen vegetables may cost more than fresh vegetables, but they are easy to heat and eat. Since they are quickly frozen after harvest, they retain their vitamins. If the fresh vegetables don't seem to be a good buy, check out the frozen ones.

Healthy food is expensive. I try to buy only what-
ever is necessary. Fruits are expensive. In fact, every-
thing is expensive, especially the healthy foods.
                                        Carlota, 18 – Luis, 41/2

If you can get to a farmer's market, you can probably find fresher and less expensive fruits and vegetables. The **<www.mypyramid.gov>** website has a list of farmer's markets across the country. After you put in your personal information (age and sex), click the submit button.

Click on the Tips section of the Fruits block for this information. Go to "Buy fresh fruits in season," and click. You'll find "Find a Farmers Market in Your State." Click on it for the possible location of a farmer's market near you.

Some people prefer to buy organic foods, i.e., foods

grown without use of pesticides or other unnecessary chemicals. Usually organic foods are more expensive, although at a farmers market this may not be so. If yu can afford them, organically produced dairy products are a good choice.

Tips for Buying Meat

I get WIC and they provide me with milk, cereal, and juices. So what I have to buy is the meat, chicken, the main dishes, rice. I don't spend as much as I thought I would because WIC provides a lot of help. Sometimes they have coupons for Farmers Market.

Ukari

Meat is one of the more expensive items on your grocery list. Cuts of beef vary a lot. Round is tougher, but has a good flavor for many things. Round and less expensive roasts are good when slowly cooked with sauce and seasonings in a pot or crock-pot.

If you can afford it, look for ground beef with a fat content of 10 to 15 percent. Ground meat with higher fat content is not very good for you or your family.

If you find a reasonable price, buy fresh ground beef in

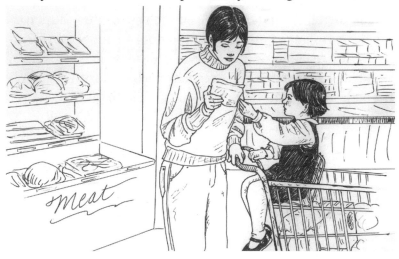

preference to pre-packaged. The quality and condition is likely to be better. Always cook ground meat thoroughly.

Pork, Poultry, and Fish

Center cut pork chops have a good flavor but they cost more. Tenderloin is a very tender cut but expensive. End chops and shoulder taste good, but you need more time and patience to trim out the tough connective tissue and fat. This meat is good for stir-fry once it is trimmed out.

Back strips, if you can find them, may be the least expensive. This is a top quality cut and easy to cook.

Ham is often quite cheap in the winter and spring near holidays. Turkeys also tend to be a good buy near the holidays in the fall and winter.

Chicken is usually less expensive than beef, and buying a whole chicken is generally cheaper than a package of precut breasts, legs, and thighs.

Fish should be a part of a healthy diet. Fish is high in protein and low in saturated fats, and they contain important fatty acids. As mentioned before, the risk of mercury contamination is highest in swordfish, shark, king mackerel and tilefish, although all fish contains some mercury.

Choose other kinds of seafood such as shrimp, salmon, tilapia, catfish and canned light tuna. As mentioned before, it's *okay* to eat two or three servings of these fish weekly.

Neither fresh nor defrosted fish keeps well for very long. If you have any question about the condition of the fish, don't eat it. Uncooked fish spoils easily.

Two-Family Households

I live with my husband's parents. We cook on our own part of the time, and eat with them part of the time. Generally my husband and Kendall and I eat together, but not the others.

Sometimes the other kids want some of our food

and I don't have enough. I give them some because I
feel bad if I don't. It's kind of hard because I only have
enough money to buy for our family. And sometimes
they get into my refrigerator.

I try not to say anything because I don't want to
get into an argument with his mom. Sometimes my
daughter does the same — gets into their stuff, and I
tell her she shouldn't. For the most part, they know
how to respect my stuff.

It's hard to share a home and try to buy food. I
have my own refrigerator and they have theirs, and
we each have a microwave.

Ukari

Living with another family brings added complications.
Does each person or parent/child buy their own food? How
do they keep it separate? At least Ukari has her own refrigerator. If everything is in one refrigerator, families usually
designate a particular shelf or shelves for each family unit.

If each family unit cooks for themselves, a schedule
for kitchen use may help. Or perhaps adults will take turns
cooking for the entire family. You may do some experiment-
ing before you find a system that works best for all of you.

Your Toddler Can Help

Let your toddler help you shop. Be sure he's seated
securely in the basket of the grocery cart. Let him hold an
unbreakable item or two – perhaps a bag of carrots or can
of refried beans. He may be interested in helping you cook
some of the food you're buying. See chapter 11 for recipes
to use with a child.

What choices can you give him as you shop? Can he
decide whether you'll buy grapes or mangos? Chicken or
ground beef? He's likely to be enthusiastic about eating the
good food he helps you buy. *What a team you are!*

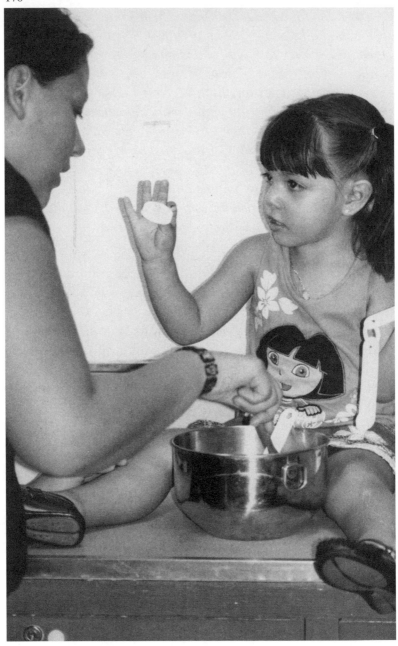

She loves to help Mom cook.

11

Cooking with Mom

- **Let Him Help**
- **Focus on Safety**
- **Snacks to Prepare Together**
- **Quick Meals for Kids**
- **Main Dishes She Can Help Prepare**
- **Notes About Cheese**
- **He Can Help with Desserts Too**
- **Eating for Health and Pleasure**

Andrea cooks with me all the time. She's our little Betty Crocker. She has her own apron that she decorated and her own step stool. She really knows her way around the kitchen.

We're always eating bananas. Andrea likes to fix them. First, she crushes the nuts. We put them in a bag and she mashes them with a rolling pin.

Then she peels the banana and rolls it in the nuts. She loves to cook.

Vanesa, 19 – Andrea, 4; Josefina, 8 months

Let Him Help

Even a toddler can help mom or dad in the kitchen. He can wash the lettuce and the fruit. In fact, you'll think of all sorts of ways he can help you "cook."

The following recipes include several that are mostly doable by a toddler, such as the recipe for bean dip. Of course you'll organize ingredients and provide whatever help he needs.

As he matures, he can do more and more of these recipes mostly by himself. Is he a picky eater? Most children want to eat what they prepare themselves.

Always make it fun. He's not old enough yet to take over the cooking or to cook on demand. Cooking with mom or dad, however, can be a great bonding experience for everyone involved. It can also be lots of fun:

> *For one of the parties we had, we made scenery out of vegetables – broccoli for trees, on a paper plate. The kids did their own paper plates.*
>
> *You paint the trunks brown with edible paint, paint the grapes brown for rocks, peas into little pebbles. One kid made a dinosaur out of the grapes, and the string bean was the tail.*
>
> *When the paint dries, it kind of holds it together like it was glue.*
>
> Vanesa

If you are a neatnik, you may have to take a deep breath and relax — children are usually pretty messy when they're cooking.

As the years go by, you'll teach him to clean up the messes he makes because that's part of cooking. For now, he'll often be willing to help with the cleanup, if he considers it fun.

Letting toddlers and preschoolers cook will not make

your work easier. Of course you could prepare these dishes faster by yourself, but that's not the point. It's important for your child's development that he is able to work with you when he wants to.

Focus on Safety

Safety is an important issue.

Children under three should probably not cook anything hot. They can watch the procedure and help prepare the ingredients, but you should do the actual cooking.

Preschoolers learn best when cooking something quickly, such as scrambled eggs. They can also use the toaster to make toast, but make sure they don't *touch the toaster*.

It's best to begin with solid foods (such as the eggs) because liquids spread so quickly when spilled. Hot liquids can cause a burn on a large part of a young child's body.

Your child can be deciding what to make, help you make a list, shop with you. She can wash fruits and vegetables. She can get out the measuring cups and spoons, etc. All of these are safe for a child of any age as long as there are no glass items involved. Children under five should not be using the electric mixer. Even after that age they need to be closely supervised.

Mackenzie helps in the kitchen every day. She's a list girl. First, we make a list of everything we need, and she'll get out this big giant bowl. I read the list and she finds everything. Then we start mixing.

Normally we start by cutting up the vegetables. We have this child-safe knife that's meant for lettuce, but she uses it for everything. It's plastic.

She helps me cut up stuff. She helps me measure — which I think is good because she gets some math in there. And off we go.

*I never let her do anything with the oven or
the stove.*

Hannah, 23 — Mackenzie, 41/2

Be sure that all "cooks" wash their hands before starting.
Children love to lick the spoons and scrapers used in cooking. What fun! Just be sure the same spoon or scraper does
not go back into the food you're preparing. Children with
coughs and runny noses shouldn't be involved in the food
preparation. Perhaps they can set the table instead.

Beginning knife use is safer with the plastic knives that
come with fast food or that you can buy in small boxes at
the grocery store. They have rounded tips and are serrated
(have a jagged edge) for easier cutting.

If you should have a fire in the kitchen while you're
cooking, the best advice is to cover it quickly and turn off
the heat. Move yourself and your child away from the
danger and call 911 if you need help.

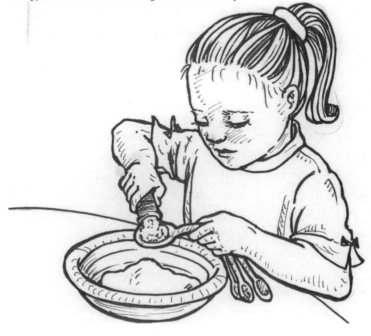

Do not leave the house while something is cooking. The only exception is the slow cooker which is intended to cook for a long time at a slow heat. Follow the directions for the cooker.

Bring the phone into the kitchen before you begin cooking so you don't have to leave the room. Never leave your child unattended in the kitchen, even for a few minutes.

If she stirs anything on the stove, be sure you're right there beside her. You know your child, so you can figure out her safety issues.

She needs a very sturdy stool to stand on while she's working at your kitchen counter. Or she can work at the kitchen table using a booster seat or high chair. She may want to help with the dishes, and will need her stool.

> *Mackenzie does my dishes. I wash them, and she rinses them and stacks them in the drying racks. We use regular dishes, and she's been doing it for about a year.*
>
> *She's like my little Cinderella. She'll ask, "Can I clean the floor?"*
>
> *I say, "Yes, go ahead," and she sings a Cinderella song while she does it.*
>
> *She always asks for things to do. I think a lot of people don't have the time — sometimes it takes a little more time than if I did it myself, but that's okay.*
>
> Hannah

Snacks to Prepare Together
Cauliflower Posies

1 teaspoon olive oil   **2 teaspoons butter**
Cauliflower, cut up like flowers

Put olive oil and butter in a Teflon®-coated skillet. Use all olive oil if you prefer. Cut the cauliflower up like flowers, and stir-fry.

Mackenzie's Smoothie

What we do a lot is like at mid-morning, at 11 we make a smoothie. First, you have to have a real good blender. We have a good smoothie every day.

My blender never gets put away. We use it probably more than once a day. It's a permanent fixture on our counter. The smoothie is easy. Mackenzie can practically do it herself.

**Plain yogurt   Small amount of juice
Any kind of fruits you like**.

Cut up the fruit, like fresh strawberries. We throw that all in. Sometimes we throw in some ice cubes.

Sometimes I'm taking a shower, and I'll come out and Mackenzie will say, "Mom, I have all the stuff in the blender."

I say, "Don't push the button yet," and she says "OK."

It's easy, very little mess. I empty the blender, put a little soap and water in it, turn it on, and it's clean.

Hannah

Bean Dip

**1/3 cup canned refried beans
Grated cheddar cheese
Chips or crackers**

Get out a shallow bowl. Place approximately 1/3 cup canned refried beans in the bowl. Use a fork to flatten beans along bottom of bowl. If playing is more important than hunger, this may take a while.

Sprinkle with grated cheddar cheese. Microwave on high for 45 seconds. Remove, place a circle of chips or crackers around the edge in the dip to make it look like a flower.

Multipurpose Trail Mix

**1 cup whole-wheat cereal (Life®, Cheerios®, or
   Chex®)**
1 cup pretzels, broken into small pieces
**1/4 cup pine nuts, sliced almonds or sunflower
   seeds**
1/2 cup rice cracker mix
**Optional: raisins, chopped dried apricots,
   or dried cranberries**

Pour everything in a large bowl. Mix together. Store
in a sealed container or large zip bag. Place a quarter-cup
measuring cup in the container or bag. If you're in a hurry,
put 1/4 cup for a toddler or 1/2 cup for a preschooler in a
small plastic bag. With a non-spill cup of milk this is a great
breakfast on the go. It is also great to have along if you are
shopping.

Try different combinations of ingredients. Let your child
do the mixing and selecting. Add dried fruit such as raisins,
chopped dried apricots or dried cranberries after you scoop
up the dry ingredients. (If you mix these in ahead of time,
the mixture gets soggy.)

Vanesa's Trail Mix

*We do a lot of hiking and fishing and we make trail
mix to take along. I have a dehydrator, and we use
nuts, cranberries, raisins, bananas, strawberries, kiwi,
mainly fruit.*

Vanesa

Moon Balls

1/3 cup peanut butter   2/3 cup dry milk or Nido
1/3 cup honey

Mix together and form into balls. Don't give to child
under a year because of the honey.

Quick Crispy Snack
1 whole wheat pita bread   1/2 cup hummus*

Heat oven to 350°.

Cut the pita bread in 8 triangles. Split each triangle. Put pieces on cookie sheet in a single layer. Put in oven for 10 minutes. Put hummus on small plate with toasted pita chips around it. Enjoy!

*Hummus is a bean dip made from garbanzo beans. If you can't find it, use bean dip or salsa. This is also good with **low-fat sour cream with chopped pine nuts.**

Pretzels

This is a popular recipe among all ages of kids and can be done in an hour. Encourage children to make pretzels in various shapes. Let their imaginations take over. Perhaps they'll even make some in animal shapes.

1 package yeast
11/2 cups warm water
1 tablespoon sugar
4 cups flour
1 egg, beaten and set aside
1 tablespoon salt
Pretzel or coarse salt
Oil spray

In a big bowl mix together yeast, water, sugar and salt. Stir in the flour. Place on floured table or bread board and knead until dough is smooth. Shape the dough into pretzel shapes (using imagination).

Set on tray sprayed with oil or lined with parchment paper. Brush with beaten egg. Sprinkle with coarse salt.

Bake in 425° oven for 15 minutes or until browned.

Serve with cheese dip or mustard.

Toasted Pumpkin Seeds

Take seeds from a big pumpkin. In a bowl of warm water, clean off all the slimy strings. Put the seeds on a towel to drain. Move them to a baking sheet, and toast in a 350° oven until crisp. Delicious snack, high in protein and minerals.

Quick Meals for Kids

Suggestions for quick snacks and lunches:

- Peanut butter and jelly sandwiches, grilled or not

- Peanut butter on crackers

- Grilled cheese sandwich on whole wheat bread, tortillas, or English muffins with fresh veggies or fruit

- Quesadilla (Put cheese between two tortillas. Heat in skillet, grill, or oven.)

- Macaroni and cheese or spaghetti with peas

- Dry tortellini cooked with ready-made spaghetti sauce. Throw in some fresh tomato, grated carrot or green beans for a meal in one.

- Try various shapes of pasta. There are often some in the market with holiday themes.

- Yogurt with cereal and fruit

- English muffin pizza

- Apples with peanut butter

- Quick snacks
    - √ popcorn (not for toddlers — choking risk)
    - √ dry cereal
    - √ nuts with raisins
    - √ frozen peas

Do you have somebody who doesn't like sandwiches? You might try cutting off the crust. If you aren't using the crusts for croutons or poultry stuffing, toss it outside for the birds.

Leanne's Applesauce Sun
Applesauce
Thin slices of American cheese
Raisins

Prepare shallow dish of applesauce, surrounded by thin slices of American cheese for rays. Make a happy face with raisins.

Generally speaking, kids love happy faces and hearts on or with their foods. You can pick up assorted heart shaped bowls and plates cheaply at your local thrift store.

Leanne loves to pour her own beverages just like in Montessori school. You can find a variety of inexpensive small pitchers and creamers at thrift stores for your child.

Betty Sue, 18 - Leanne, 4

Rachel's Scrambled Eggs
Kylie loves helping me fix scrambled eggs. He likes to get out the stuff, and he can help me stir when I'm right there.

Rachel, 19 – Kylie, 41/2; Terry, 2

Make scrambled eggs with grated carrots, a few peas, or any leftover cooked vegetable. Let your preschooler stir the eggs (with your constant supervision).

Make a design with the veggies. Grated cheese makes great hair to top off a veggie "face."

Main Dishes She Can Help Prepare

Andrea's Ham and Cheese Loaf

1 pound frozen pizza dough
1 8-ounce package deli ham or turkey
1 cup shredded cheddar cheese
1/4 cup mayonnaise   1 beaten egg
1 tablespoon grated Parmesan cheese

Set oven at 350°. Place thawed dough on lightly floured surface. Flatten with hands. Roll into a rectangle with rolling pin.

Top evenly with ham, leaving 1/2" border around all sides. Mix cheddar cheese and mayonnaise and spread over ham. Moisten edges of dough with water.

Starting at one of the long sides of dough, fold one-third of the dough over the filling. Then repeat with other long side of dough. Firmly pinch edge of dough together to seal.

Place seam side down on lightly greased baking sheet. Cut diagonal slits in top of dough. Brush evenly with egg. Sprinkle the Parmesan cheese on it.

Bake 35-40 minutes until golden brown. Cool 10 minutes before cutting. Cut into slices.

Andrea does most of this ham and cheese loaf. She really knows her way around the kitchen. She has her own apron that she decorated and her own step stool.

Vanesa

Holiday Dinner Rolls

For all holidays we get the frozen bread dough, thaw, and shape for the current holiday (Valentine hearts, Thanksgiving turkeys, Christmas trees, etc.). This is a fun family activity. Follow directions on package after shaping.

Betty Sue

Evelyn's Lasagna

If you are using mushrooms you might have your child begin to chop them here using a non-serrated utensil knife with rounded tip. Josephine has always been in charge of chopping the mushrooms. She loves to do it and, perhaps because of some basic safety reviews, she has never hurt herself.

1 (261/2-oz.) can or jar of spaghetti sauce
1/2 can water

Heat oven to 350°.

Heat above ingredients in a saucepan. Supplement as desired, perhaps with one or more of the following:

1/2 cup chopped red peppers
1 cup sliced mushrooms   Other vegetables
1/2 teaspoon anise seed   Cooked meat

Prepare cheese filling in large bowl:

2 cups low fat cottage cheese (half may be part-skim ricotta)
2 cups shredded low fat mozzarella cheese
1 teaspoon garlic   1/8 teaspoon black pepper

You can also add two cups cooked vegetables such as spinach or broccoli to the cheese mixture.

Build lasagna in a 10" x 14" baking dish as follows:

Cover bottom of the dish with half the sauce. Then arrange a layer of uncooked lasagna on top of the sauce. Cover that with all the cheese filling.

Place second layer of lasagna in the dish. Cover it with remaining sauce. Be sure all pasta is covered by the sauce. (Quantity of sauce will vary due to choice of vegetable additions. If there is not enough sauce, just add some water.) Sprinkle with Parmesan cheese. Cover with foil.

Bake 40-55 minutes.

Bread Pizza

Hard roll or English muffin split open
Spaghetti sauce or pizza sauce
Shredded cheese of your choice: mozzarella,
cheddar, jack
Toppings of your choice: tomatoes, mushrooms,
onions, pepperoni slices

Heat broiler.

Ask your child to place the roll on a cookie sheet. Spread sauce on the top, then sprinkle with cheese and topping. Broil 2+ minutes as needed.

Notes About Cheese

Cheese is often a popular food because of its flavor and convenience. Young children like it, and children's menus in restaurants often feature cheese either grilled or with macaroni. Because a young child eats small amounts, it is a good source of both protein for strength and brain development and a substitute for milk when milk is not available or the child is not interested in milk for a while.

However, in adult portions, cheese is high in fat and in sodium. Both of these items cause weight gain and can disturb the balance in your good eating pattern if you use them too often.

As mentioned in chapter 1, the healthiest cheese for a pregnant woman is low-fat cottage cheese or ricotta cheese. Mozzarella cheese is somewhat lower in fat and sodium, but should be used moderately. This and all cheeses are higher than 30 percent fat unless you buy the non-fat kind.

So when you eat regular cheese, be sure to round your meal out with items low in fat and sodium like vegetables and fruits as well as whole grain breads, pasta, tortillas, or pita.

He Can Help with Desserts Too

You know how you can get those concentrated fruit drinks? We make popsicles with those in ice trays.

We make Jell-O in the regular way, then put fruit like dried cranberries in half of it. Then we put the rest of the Jell-O on top.

If you can cook things in different ways, I think kids will eat it.

Like beans, if you find a way she really likes them, then you give her a dried up old cookie, there's no comparison.

                                                    Vanesa

Granita

This is a fun summertime treat. It's easy to make, has no fat, and tastes like a sno-cone. Be sure you will be home for a while when making this one.

1 cup water
1/3 cup sugar
2 cups of your favorite fruit

Put the fruit in the blender and puree until it is thin like soup.

Put the water and sugar in a small pan and cook for 5 minutes.

Add the fruit to the sugar water and stir up.

Pour into a flat metal pan. (A 9" x 13" cake pan works well.)

Put into freezer.

Every 30 minutes, rake the mixture with a fork. Do this three times. Then put it into a bowl and put back in the freezer for one hour.

Take out and put into bowls. Enjoy!

Instant Pudding
This can be very rewarding for a first cooking experi-
ence. Your child can do it all by herself. Ask her to get a
bowl, open the package, pour it into the bowl. She'll need a
few minutes to play in the pudding mix.

1 package instant pudding mix
2 cups milk

Add one cup milk and stir thoroughly to avoid tricky
lumps before adding the second cup. She can use a variety
of stirrers such as a whisk, fork, or spoon. Follow the
directions on the package.

If you're concerned about making a mess, you may want
to stick to vanilla pudding. Perhaps she could sprinkle the
finished pudding with chocolate chips when she serves it.

Cowboy Cookies
This has been a family favorite for a few generations. It's
a great recipe because most of the measurements are full
cups that are easy for a child to handle. They learn to fluff
the flour, push down on the brown sugar, then level off with
a knife/edge.

Josephine usually has her own work area where she is
comfortable measuring things out over a flexible mat. This
makes it easy to pour the overflow back in the container.

1 cup butter	**1 cup sugar**
1 cup brown sugar	**2 eggs**
1 teaspoon vanilla	**1 1/2 cups flour**
1/2 cup whole wheat flour	**1/2 t. baking powder**
1/2 teaspoon salt	**1 t. baking soda**
2 cups oats	**1 cup chocolate chips**

Blend butter, sugars, eggs, and vanilla. Add dry ingredients. Mix well. Add oats and chips. Bake on greased sheets.
350°, 8-10 minutes. Makes 5 dozen.

Eating for Health and Pleasure

Throughout these chapters, we have tried to present sound ideas and suggestions for you and your child to develop healthy eating habits. This is important, of course, but we know that simply eating the same foods day after day gets old.

This can be true regarding fast foods, too. No matter how much you like French fries, soda, and super-size hamburgers, you may be surprised at the pleasure good healthy food can provide.

This is why we have encouraged you to serve a wide variety of appetizing and healthy foods to your child and the rest of your family. We know this is essential for optimal health. We also think you will discover that healthy food can taste mighty good!

Enjoy your meal planning, food shopping, cooking (sometimes with your child helping), and especially enjoy the good food you serve. *You can make life more satisfying for you and your family.*

Bibliography

The following bibliography contains books, websites, and journal references of interest to young parents. Prices are quoted for the books, but because prices change so rapidly, call your local or Internet book store or your local library reference department for an updated price and address before ordering a book. See pages 195-196 for an order form for Morning Glory Press publications.

Andrews, Sam S., M.D., et al. *Sugar Busters! for Kids.* 2001. 220 pp. $23.95. Ballantine Books.
Presents good articles against fast food and sweets, especially soft drinks, french fries, candy, and sugar-coated cereals.

González, M.D. *My Child Won't Eat! How to Prevent and Solve the Problem.* 2005. 183 pp. $12.95. La Leche League International.
Good discussion of feeding babies on demand — including not pushing solid foods as well as breast or bottle. Baby knows best!

Kalnins, Daina, and Joanne Saab. *Better Baby Food: Your Essential Guide to Nutrition, Feeding and Cooking for Your Baby and Toddler.* 2001. 256 pp. $18.95. Robert Rose Pub.

*Information on general infant nutrition, breastfeeding, formulas, and baby's
first solid foods. Recipes for breakfast, lunch, dinner, snacks, and desserts for
children from six months through 18 months.*

_____. ***Better Food for Kids: Your Essential Guide to Nutrition for
all Children from Age 2 to 6.*** 2002. 256 pp. $17.95. Robert Rose
Pub.
*Includes health and nutrition information as well as recipes. Discusses tips
for feeding picky eaters.*

La Leche League International. ***The Womanly Art of Breastfeeding:
Seventh Revised Edition.*** 2004. 480 pp. $18.00. Plume.
*For almost fifty years mothers who have been in touch with La Leche League
have found the kind of information and support they need to breastfeed their
babies. This book offers the same kind of help.*

Lansky, Vickie, and Kathy Rogers. ***Feed Me — I'm Yours***. 2004. 143
pp. $10. Meadowbrook, Inc.
*An excellent cookbook for new parents. Lots of recipes for making baby food
"from scratch." Also includes directions for kitchen crafts.*

_____. ***Taming of the C.A.N.D.Y. Monster: Continuously Advertised
Nutritionally Deficient Yummies: A Cookbook.*** 1999. 165 pp. $9.95.
Book Peddlers.
*Practical, easy-to-make, and delicious recipes. Contains concise, humorous,
and informative passages and tried and true food ideas.*

Leach, Penelope. ***Your Baby and Child from Birth to Age Five.***
Revised, 1997. 560 pp. $20. Alfred A. Knopf.
*An absolutely beautiful book packed with information, many color photos
and lovely drawings. Comprehensive, authoritative, and outstandingly
sensitive guide to nutrition, child care and development.*

Lindsay, Jeanne Warren. ***The Challenge of Toddlers*** and ***Your Baby's
First Year (Teens Parenting*** **Series).** 2004. 224 pp. each.   Paper,
$12.95 each; cloth, $18.95 each. Morning Glory Press. 888.612.8254.
*How-to-parent books especially for teenage parents. Lots of quotes from
teenage parents who share their experiences. Includes chapters on feeding
babies and toddlers.* ***Your Baby's First Year*** *is available in regular, Easier
Reading, and Spanish (**El primer año del bebé**) editions.*

_____. ***Teenage Couples — Coping with Reality: Dealing with
Money, In-laws, Babies and Other Details of Daily Life.*** 1995. 192
pp. Paper, $9.95. Morning Glory Press.
*Along with the practical details of living, it includes a chapter on food
shopping and budgeting. Lots of quotes from teenage couples.*

_____. ***Teen Dads: Rights, Responsibilities and Joys (Teens***

Parenting **Series)**. 2001. 224 pp. $12.95. Morning Glory Press.
A how-to-parent book especially for teenage fathers. Offers help in parenting from conception to age three of the child, including feeding information. Many quotes from and photos of teen fathers. For detailed teaching help, see **Teen Dads Comprehensive Curriculum Notebook** *($125 ea.).*

_____ and Jean Brunelli. *Nurturing Your Newborn: Young Parent's Guide to Baby's First Month.* (*Teens Parenting* **Series***)* 2005. 96 pp. $7.95. Available in regular, Easier Reading, and Spanish (*Crianza del recién nacido)* editions. Morning Glory Press.
Focuses on the postpartum period. Ideal for teen parents home after delivery. For detailed teaching help, see **Nurturing Your Newborn/Your Baby's First Year Comprehensive Curriculum Notebook ($125).**

_____, _____ . *Your Pregnancy and Newborn Journey (Teens Parenting* **Series).** 2004. 224 pp. Paper, $12.95; cloth, $18.95; Regular, Spanish (*Tu embarazo y el nacimiento de tu bebé),* and Easier Reading edition. Morning Glory Press.
Prenatal health book for pregnant teens. Includes section on breastfeeding, care of the newborn, and chapter for fathers.

_____ and Sally McCullough. *Discipline from Birth to Three.* 2004. 224 pp. Paper, $12.95; cloth, $18.95. Morning Glory Press.
Provides teenage parents with guidelines to help prevent discipline problems with children, and for dealing with problems when they occur.

MELD Parenting Materials. **Nueva Familia.** Six books, each in Spanish and English editions. *Baby Is Here. Feeding Your Child, 5 months-2 years. Healthy Child, Sick Child. Safe Child and Emergencies. Baby Grows. Baby Plays.* 1992. $12 each. MELD, Suite 507, 123 North Third Street, Minneapolis, MN 55401. 612.332.7563.
Very easy to read books full of information. Designed especially for Mexican and Mexican American families, but excellent for anyone with limited reading skills. Ask MELD for catalog of other materials designed especially for school-age parents.

Renfrew, Mary, Chloe Fisher, and Suzanne Arms. *Bestfeeding: Getting Breastfeeding Right for You.* 2004. 296 pp. $17.95. Ten Speed Press.
Marvelous description, with lots of photographs and drawings (150+) of the importance of breastfeeding, and of how to make the process work.

Sears, Martha and William. *The Breastfeeding Book: Everything You Need to Know About Nursing Your Child from Birth Through Weaning.* 2000. 272 pp. $14.99. Little, Brown.
Discusses, among other topics, the practical challenges of breastfeeding that confront many women who work away from home.

Shulman, Martha Rose, M.D., and Jane Davis. *Every Woman's Guide to Eating During Pregnancy.* 2002. 288 pp. $16.00. Houghton Mifflin.
Includes 100 recipes framed in a crash course on nutrition. Basic tips on weight gain, bed rest, fighting nausea, key nutrients, and other issues are discussed.

Walker, W. Allan., and Courtney Humphries. *The Harvard Medical School Guide to Healthy Eating During Pregnancy.* 2005. 304 pp. $16.95. McGraw-Hill.
Offers a great deal of solid information and medically sound advice on prenatal nutrition.

Wiggins, Pamela K. *Why Should I Nurse My Baby?* 1998. 58 pp. $5.95. Noodle Soup, 4614 Prospect Avenue, #328, Cleveland, OH 44103. 216.881.5151.
Easy-to-read, yet thorough discussion of breastfeeding.

Young, Nicole, and Nadine Day. *Blender Baby Food: Over 125 Recipes for Healthy Homemade Meals.* 2005. 192 pp. $18.95. Robert Rose.
Simple recipes that make it easy to make baby's food at home.

Websites
All sites begin with www.

aap.org – **American Academy of Pediatrics**. Provides reliable information on many topics regarding child health and development.

acog.org – **American College of Obstetricians and Gynecologists.** Information about pregnancy and breastfeeding.

ada.org – **American Dental Association.** Good for information on nutrition, health, and dental health.

americandieteticassociation.org – Information on current dietary recommendations, gestational diabetes, fat and sodium recommendations. Also has site **eatright.org** for standards on child care nutrition.

arbys.com – Nutrition information on foods served here.

dairyqueen.com – Nutrition information on foods served at this chain.

elpolloloco.com – Nutrition information on foods served at this restaurant.

usda.gov – **U.S. Department of Agriculture**. Wealth of information including **MyPyramid** for all ages.

futureofchildren.org – **Packard Foundation** site has timely publication regarding current research on many topics around children.

kfc.com – Information on dietary values of food served here.

lungoregon.org/tobacco/secondhand.html – Discussion of risks of inhaling second-hand smoke.

mcdonalds.com/app_controller.nutrition.Index1.html – Complete nutrition information on all foods served at McDonald's restaurants.

mypyramid.gov – **U.S. Department of Agriculture.** Put in your age, sex, and activity level, and you'll get a chart showing the foods *you* need. Do the same for your child 2 years or older.

nlm.nih.gov/medlineplus – **National Institutes of Health** site for reliable source of dietary information.

nrc.uchsc.edu – **National Resource Center for Health and Safety in Child Care and Early Education.**

pizzahut.com – Another site for specific nutrition information.

tacobell.com – Nutrition information from this restaurant.

Most fast food restaurants have web sites and/or handouts available at their local restaurants. Dine-in restaurants may not have either since their menu varies greatly and their foods are prepared on site by individual chefs. Fast food franchises have a set menu and deliver foods to local sites ready to serve as offered.

Periodicals

Hauck, Fern R, Omojokun, Olanrewaju O., Siadaty, Mir S., *Pediatrics*, November, 2005, Vol. 116, pgs. 716-723, **"Do Pacifiers Reduce the Risk of S.I.D.S.? A Meta-Analysis."**

Kumanyika, S, Grier, S., *Future of Children*, Spring, 2006, Vol 16, No. l, pgs. 187-207. **"Targeting Interventions for Ethnic Minority and Low-Income Populations."**

Story, M., Kaphingst, K, and French, S., *Future of Children*, Vol. 16, No. 1, Spring, 2006, pgs. 143-168. **"The Role of Child Care Sttings in Obesity Prevention."**

"Obesity's Heavy Burden." *UCLA Public Health*, June, 2006, pp. 6-11.

About the Authors

Jeanne Warren Lindsay, Jean Brunelli, and Sally McCullough worked together for many years at Tracy High School, Cerritos, California. Jeanne founded and directed the Teen Parent Program for 16 years. Sally was the head teacher at the Tracy Infant Center, while Jean was the Infant Center nurse. Sally and Jean each served several years as director of the Handicapped Infant Program at the same school. Jean also taught a weekly prenatal health class in Jeanne's program.

Jean is the co-author, with Jeanne, of *Your Pregnancy and Newborn Journey* and *Nurturing Your Newborn.* Sally co-authored, with Jeanne, *Discipline from Birth to Three.* Each provided input into Jeanne's other books for pregnant and parenting teens.

Jean is a PHN and a graduate of Mount St. Mary's College, Los Angeles. She and Mike have two grown children and three grandchildren.

Sally's academic degree is in psychology, but her practical experience, professionally and personally, has made her an expert on child-rearing. She and Stuart have three children and five grandchildren.

Jeanne's education includes an M.A. in home economics and an M.A. in anthropology, each with an emphasis on child development. She and Bob have five children and seven grandchildren.

All three authors live in the Los Angeles area.

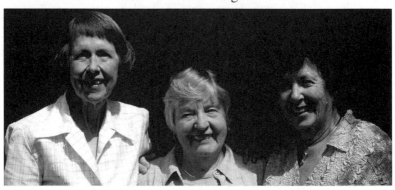

Sally McCullough, Jeanne Lindsay, Jean Brunelli

Index

Morning Glory Press
6595 San Haroldo Way, Buena Park, CA 90620
714.828.1998; 888.612.8254   Fax 1.888.327.4362
Contact us for complete catalog including quantity and other discounts.

	Price	Total
__ **Complete** *Teens Parenting* **Curriculum**	$1208.00	_____

One each — Six *Comprehensive Curriculum Notebooks*
plus 9 books, 7 workbooks, 8 videos/DVDs, 5 games
(Everything on this page of order form)
Buy a text and workbook for each student.
Contact us for generous quantity discounts.

Resources for Teen Parent Teachers/Counselors:

	Price	Total
__ *Books, Babies and School-Age Parents*	14.95	_____
__ *ROAD to Fatherhood*	14.95	_____

Resources for Teen Parents:

	Price	Total
__ *Mommy, I'm Hungry!* Quality paper	12.95	_____
__ *Mommy, I'm Hungry!* Hardcover	18.95	_____
__ *Mommy, I'm Hungry! Curriculum Notebook*	125.00	_____
__ *Your Pregnancy and Newborn Journey*	12.95	_____
__ **Easier Reading Edition (GL2)**	12.95	_____
__ *Tu embarazo y el nacimiento de tu bebé*	12.95	_____
__ *PNJ Curriculum Notebook*	125.00	_____
__ **PNJ Board Game**	29.95	_____
__ *Pregnancy Two-in-One Bingo*	19.95	_____
__ *Nurturing Your Newborn*	7.95	_____
__ **Easier Reading Edition (GL2)**	7.95	_____
__ *Crianza del recién nacido*	7.95	_____
__ *Your Baby's First Year*	12.95	_____
__ **Easier Reading Edition (GL2)**	12.95	_____
__ *El primer año del bebé*	12.95	_____
__ *BFY/NN Curriculum Notebook*	125.00	_____
__ **Four Videos/DVDs – Baby's First Year Series**	195.00	_____
__ **Baby's First Year Board Game**	29.95	_____
__ *Discipline from Birth to Three*	12.95	_____
__ *Discipline Curriculum Notebook*	125.00	_____
__ **Four Videos/DVDs– Discipline Birth to Three Series**	195.00	_____
__ **Discipline from Birth to Three Board Game**	29.95	_____
__ *The Challenge of Toddlers*	12.95	_____
__ *CT Curriculum Notebook*	125.00	_____
__ **Challenge of Toddlers Board Game**	29.95	_____
__ *Teen Dads: Rights, Responsibilities and Joys*	12.95	_____
__ *Teen Dads Curriculum Notebook*	125.00	_____
SUBTOTAL (Carry over to top of next page.)		_____

SUBTOTAL FROM PREVIOUS PAGE   _____

More Resources for Teen Parents:

Following books are NOT included in Complete *Teens Parenting* Curriculum:

__ *Moving On*	4.95	_____
__ *Will the Dollars Stretch?*	7.95	_____
__ *Dreams to Reality: Help for Young Moms*	14.95	_____
__ *Do I Have a Daddy?* Hardcover	14.95	_____
__ *Goodnight, Daddy* Hardcover	14.95	_____
__ *Did My First Mother Love Me?* Hardcover	12.95	_____
__ *Pregnant? Adoption Is an Option*	12.95	_____
__ *Surviving Teen Pregnancy*	12.95	_____
__ *Safer Sex: The New Morality*	14.95	_____
__ *Teen Moms: The Pain and the Promise*	14.95	_____
__ *Teenage Couples: Caring, Commitment and Change*	9.95	_____
— *Teenage Couples: Coping with Reality*	9.95	_____

Novels by Marilyn Reynolds:

__ *Love Rules*	9.95	_____
__ *If You Loved Me*	8.95	_____
__ *Baby Help*	8.95	_____
__ *But What About Me?*	8.95	_____
__ *Too Soon for Jeff*	8.95	_____
__ *Detour for Emmy*	8.95	_____
__ *Telling*	8.95	_____
__ *Beyond Dreams*	8.95	_____

SUBTOTAL   _____

Add postage: 10% of total—Min., $3.50; 20%, Canada   _____

California residents add 7.75% sales tax   _____

TOTAL   _____

Ask about quantity discounts, teacher, student guides.

Prepayment requested. School/library purchase orders accepted.

NAME_____

PHONE _____   Purchase Order # _____

ADDRESS_____

_____